Holistic Approaches to Stress Management

Gabriella Goldberger

Published by Azure Time Press, 2023.

While every precaution has been taken in the preparation of this book, the publisher assumes no responsibility for errors or omissions, or for damages resulting from the use of the information contained herein.

HOLISTIC APPROACHES TO STRESS MANAGEMENT

First edition. September 7, 2023.

Copyright © 2023 Gabriella Goldberger.

ISBN: 979-8223741855

Written by Gabriella Goldberger.

Also by Gabriella Goldberger

Mindful Eating: Nourish Your Well-Being
Holistic Approaches to Stress Management
Nutrition and Immune Health
The Connection Between Sleep and Health

Table of Contents

Dedication

This book is dedicated to all those who have ever felt the weight of stress and the longing for a more balanced, peaceful life.

To every seeker of well-being who has embarked on their journey towards a healthier, happier existence – this book is for you.

To the tireless advocates of self-care, the champions of mindfulness, and the stewards of holistic living – your dedication to well-being inspires us all.

To the individuals who shared their stories of transformation and resilience, your experiences have enriched this work and serve as a beacon of hope for others.

To friends, family, and mentors who have provided unwavering support and encouragement along the way – your belief in the power of holistic well-being has been my guiding light.

May this book serve as a source of knowledge, inspiration, and practical guidance on your path to holistic stress management and lasting well-being. May you find within these pages the tools and wisdom to embrace a life of balance, vitality, and inner peace.

With gratitude and dedication,

Gabriella Goldberger

Chapter 1: Understanding Stress

Welcome to the first chapter of our journey to explore holistic approaches to managing stress. To embark on this path, it's essential to begin with a thorough understanding of stress itself – what it is, how it affects us physically and mentally, and why it's crucial to address it in our lives.

Defining Stress

Stress, in its most basic form, is your body's natural response to various demands, challenges, or threats. It's the reaction that triggers when you perceive a situation as demanding or potentially harmful. This response is deeply ingrained in our biology, dating back to our ancestors' need to survive in a world full of dangers.

Think about the last time you felt stressed. Maybe it was a tight deadline at work, a challenging exam, or a heated argument with a loved one. In these moments, your heart may have raced, your muscles tightened, and your thoughts raced. These are all common physical and emotional responses to stress.

However, it's important to understand that not all stress is harmful. In fact, some level of stress, often referred to as "eustress," can be beneficial. It can motivate you to meet deadlines, perform well in exams, or respond effectively to emergencies. Eustress is the kind of stress that keeps life exciting and helps us grow.

The Impact of Stress on Physical Health

While some stress can be positive, it's the chronic, unrelenting stress, known as "distress," that poses significant risks to our physical and mental well-being. The impact of distress on our bodies can be profound.

Imagine a scenario where you're constantly under pressure at work, juggling multiple responsibilities, and struggling to find time for relaxation. Your body interprets this prolonged stress as a threat, initiating a cascade of physiological responses. Your heart rate increases, blood pressure rises, and stress hormones like cortisol surge. Over time, this wear and tear on your body can lead to serious health problems.

High and persistent levels of stress have been linked to conditions such as hypertension (high blood pressure), cardiovascular diseases, and a weakened immune system. Chronic stress can also disrupt sleep patterns, making it difficult to get the restorative sleep you need to stay healthy.

The Impact of Stress on Mental Health

Stress doesn't limit its effects to your physical health; it can be equally detrimental to your mental well-being. When your mind is constantly preoccupied with worries and pressures, it can take a toll on your emotional stability.

Anxiety and depression often go hand in hand with chronic stress. Anxiety can manifest as excessive worry, restlessness, and a sense of impending doom, while depression may lead to persistent sadness, fatigue, and a loss of interest in once-enjoyable activities. Moreover, chronic stress can impair cognitive function, affecting your ability to think clearly and make decisions.

In essence, prolonged exposure to stress can create a vicious cycle where it not only impacts your mental health but also exacerbates physical health problems, leading to a downward spiral of well-being.

Why Understanding Stress Matters

Now that we've scratched the surface of what stress is and how it affects us, you might wonder why understanding stress matters in the first place.

Awareness is the first step toward change. By grasping the intricate ways stress operates in our lives, you gain the power to take control. You can learn to recognize the signs and symptoms of stress, identify its sources, and then take proactive steps to manage it effectively.

This book is your guide to holistic stress management, and it all begins with this understanding. In the chapters ahead, we'll explore various holistic approaches – from yoga and meditation to aromatherapy and herbal remedies – that empower you to regain control over your physical and mental well-being. These approaches offer you the tools to mitigate the harmful effects of stress, create a sense of balance, and find tranquility in the midst of life's challenges.

So, as you dive deeper into the pages of this book, remember that understanding stress is your first victory on the journey to a more relaxed and fulfilling life. It's the foundation upon which we'll build as we explore the holistic practices that will empower you to take charge of your well-being. Let's continue this exploration, one step at a time, on the path to a less stressful and more joyful life.

1. Work-Related Stressors:

For many of us, our careers are a significant source of stress. The demands of the workplace, such as tight deadlines, high expectations, and long hours, can create considerable pressure. The fear of job loss, conflicts with coworkers or superiors, and the struggle to maintain work-life balance are all common work-related stressors.

2. Financial Stressors:

Money-related stress is another prevalent issue in the modern world. Concerns about bills, debts, budgeting, and financial security can take a toll on our mental and emotional well-being. The fear of financial instability can lead to chronic anxiety and sleepless nights.

3. Relationship Stressors:

Relationships, while a source of joy, can also be a source of stress. Conflicts with partners, family members, or friends can be emotionally draining. Balancing personal and social commitments can be challenging, and navigating the complexities of human interactions can contribute to stress.

4. Technological Stressors:

The digital age has introduced a unique set of stressors. Constant connectivity through smartphones and social media can lead to information overload and a feeling of always being "on." The pressure to keep up with emails, notifications, and online expectations can be overwhelming.

5. Health-Related Stressors:

Concerns about health, both for ourselves and our loved ones, can be a significant source of stress. Worries about illness, medical bills, or maintaining a healthy lifestyle can create ongoing tension. Additionally, the prevalence of health information on the internet can lead to "cyberchondria" – excessive health-related anxiety stemming from online research.

6. Environmental Stressors:

Environmental factors, such as pollution, noise, and overcrowding, can also contribute to stress. Living in urban areas with high levels of pollution or experiencing natural disasters can trigger stress responses. These external factors can affect our well-being more than we realize.

7. Time-Related Stressors:

The modern pace of life often leads to time-related stressors. Feeling rushed, trying to fit numerous tasks into a limited timeframe, and constantly racing against the clock can elevate stress levels. This type of stress can lead to a sense of being overwhelmed and, ultimately, burnout.

8. Social and Cultural Stressors:

Societal and cultural expectations can create stress as well. Pressure to conform to certain standards, whether related to appearance, success, or lifestyle, can lead to feelings of inadequacy and stress. Discrimination and social injustices also contribute to stress, particularly for marginalized communities.

9. Traumatic Stressors:

Experiencing trauma, such as accidents, violence, or loss, can result in post-traumatic stress disorder (PTSD) and ongoing stress. The emotional aftermath of such events can have a profound impact on mental health.

10. Existential Stressors:

Questions about the purpose and meaning of life, mortality, and our place in the universe can create existential stress. These profound, philosophical concerns can lead to feelings of anxiety and unrest.

By recognizing these various stressors in modern life, you gain insight into the complexities of the challenges we face. Throughout this book, we will explore holistic approaches to manage and alleviate the impact of these stressors. Whether it's through yoga, meditation, aromatherapy, herbal remedies, or other practices, you'll find tools and guidance to navigate the diverse stressors of the modern world. The journey to a more relaxed and fulfilling life begins by understanding these stressors and equipping yourself to address them effectively.

Why Manage Stress Proactively?

Imagine your stress as a pot of water on the stove. If left unattended, it can boil over, causing damage and chaos. But if you manage it proactively, you can control the heat, preventing it from reaching a boiling point.

The same principle applies to stress in our lives. Stress, when allowed to accumulate unchecked, can have severe consequences for our physical and mental well-being. It's like a silent predator that slowly erodes our health and happiness. However, by taking a proactive approach, you can mitigate these harmful effects.

1. Preserve Your Health:

One of the most compelling reasons to manage stress proactively is to safeguard your health. Chronic stress has been linked to numerous health problems, including heart disease, hypertension, weakened immune function, and digestive issues. By actively managing stress, you reduce the risk of these health issues, ensuring a healthier and longer life.

2. Enhance Your Mental Well-being:

Proactive stress management is equally vital for your mental health. Stress can lead to anxiety, depression, and other mental health disorders. By addressing stress early on, you can maintain a positive outlook, boost your mood, and prevent the development of more severe mental health issues.

3. Improve Your Relationships:

Stress can strain your relationships with loved ones. When you're constantly on edge or overwhelmed, it's challenging to be present and nurturing in your interactions. By proactively managing stress, you can enhance your emotional well-being and improve your connections with others.

4. Boost Productivity and Creativity:

Stress often hampers productivity and stifles creativity. When your mind is preoccupied with worries, it's challenging to focus and generate innovative ideas. Managing stress proactively allows you to unleash your full potential, making you more productive and creative.

5. Enhance Your Quality of Life:

Ultimately, proactively managing stress leads to an enhanced quality of life. You'll find more joy in your daily experiences, savor moments of relaxation, and approach challenges with resilience and a sense of control. Life becomes more fulfilling when you actively steer away from chronic stress.

How to Manage Stress Proactively

So, how can you take the reins and manage stress before it takes a toll on your well-being? In the chapters ahead, we'll explore a range of holistic approaches to do just that. From yoga and meditation to aromatherapy and herbal remedies, you'll discover tools and techniques to tackle stress head-on.

But remember, proactive stress management isn't a one-size-fits-all solution. It's about finding what works best for you and integrating these practices into your daily life. It's about making a commitment to your well-being and taking small, consistent steps toward a more relaxed and fulfilling life.

In essence, this book is your guide to making proactive stress management a part of your daily routine. It's your roadmap to a healthier, happier, and more balanced life. As we journey through these holistic approaches, you'll gain the knowledge and skills to proactively address stress and reclaim control over your physical and mental well-being. So, are you ready to take that first step towards a less stressful and more fulfilling life? Let's embark on this transformative journey together.

What Is Holistic Stress Management?

Holistic stress management is an approach that recognizes the interconnectedness of the mind, body, and spirit. It acknowledges that stress affects us on multiple levels – physically, emotionally, mentally, and even spiritually. Therefore, it seeks to address stress in a comprehensive way, encompassing all these facets of our being.

In essence, holistic stress management isn't just about relieving the symptoms of stress or managing its surface-level effects. It goes beyond that. It seeks to understand the root causes of stress and offers a toolbox of practices and techniques that nurture your entire self, promoting balance, harmony, and resilience.

Why Holistic Stress Management Matters

So, why is this holistic approach to stress management so important? Well, here are a few compelling reasons:

1. Comprehensive Well-being:

Holistic stress management recognizes that true well-being isn't just the absence of stress; it's the presence of vitality, joy, and a sense of purpose. By addressing stress on all levels – physical, emotional, mental, and spiritual – it helps you cultivate a richer and more fulfilling life.

2. Sustainable Solutions:

Holistic practices are often sustainable because they focus on lifestyle changes rather than quick fixes. Instead of merely masking the symptoms of stress, these approaches encourage you to make lasting improvements that become integral parts of your daily routine.

3. Personalized Approach:

Every individual is unique, and what works for one person may not work for another. Holistic stress management allows you to tailor your approach to your specific needs and preferences, ensuring that it resonates with you on a personal level.

4. Empowerment and Self-Awareness:

Through holistic practices, you gain a deeper understanding of yourself. You become more attuned to your body's signals, your emotional responses, and your thought patterns. This self-awareness empowers you to make conscious choices that support your well-being.

5. Long-term Benefits:

By addressing stress holistically, you not only manage it effectively in the moment but also build resilience for the future. You develop the skills and habits that help you navigate life's challenges with grace and poise.

In this book, we'll explore a variety of holistic approaches to stress management, from yoga and meditation to aromatherapy and herbal remedies. Each of these practices offers a unique perspective and set of tools to help you achieve balance and calm in your life. We'll guide you through their principles, techniques, and practical applications.

But remember, holistic stress management isn't a one-time solution. It's a lifelong journey of self-discovery and self-care. It's about weaving these practices into your daily life, creating a tapestry of well-being that supports you in every moment.

So, as you continue reading, keep an open mind and an open heart. Embrace the holistic approach to stress management, knowing that it has the power to transform not only how you deal with stress but how you experience life itself. Together, we'll explore these practices and integrate them into your life, bringing you closer to a life that is relaxed, balanced, and deeply fulfilling. Are you ready to take the first step on this holistic journey? Let's begin.

1. Yoga for Stress Relief:

In the chapters dedicated to yoga, you'll discover how this ancient practice offers not only physical flexibility but also mental and emotional resilience. We'll guide you through various yoga poses and breathing exercises that can help you find calm amidst life's storms.

2. The Power of Meditation:

Meditation is more than sitting cross-legged and clearing your mind. We'll delve into mindfulness meditation, loving-kindness meditation, and other techniques that can help you quiet the mental chatter, reduce anxiety, and cultivate a sense of inner peace.

3. Aromatherapy for Stress Reduction:

Aromatherapy taps into the soothing power of scents. We'll explore how essential oils can influence your mood and relaxation. You'll learn to create your own blends and incorporate them into your daily routine for a sensory journey to tranquility.

4. Herbal Remedies and Adaptogens:

Nature provides a wealth of herbs and adaptogenic plants that can support your stress management journey. We'll discuss their benefits, how to prepare herbal remedies, and when to seek guidance from professionals for safe usage.

5. Holistic Nutrition for Stress Resilience:

Your diet plays a significant role in stress management. We'll explore how the right foods, hydration, and mindful eating can nourish not only your body but also your mind and spirit. You'll discover practical tips and holistic recipes for a balanced diet.

6. Mindful Movement and Tai Chi:

Tai Chi, a form of mindful movement, will be your gateway to gentle yet powerful practices. We'll guide you through basic Tai Chi movements and show you how this ancient art fosters relaxation, balance, and inner strength.

7. Holistic Breathwork and Pranayama:

Breathwork is the bridge between your body and mind. You'll learn various pranayama techniques, rooted in yoga traditions, to enhance your breath awareness. These exercises can be seamlessly integrated into your daily routine for moments of peace and clarity.

8. Creating Holistic Lifestyle Habits:

In this chapter, we'll discuss the importance of consistency and sustainability in holistic practices. You'll receive guidance on building a daily routine that includes holistic stress management, alongside advice on sleep, hydration, and physical activity.

9. Integrating Holistic Practices into Your Life:

As you progress through the book, you'll accumulate a toolkit of holistic practices. This chapter ties it all together, offering practical steps on how to integrate these techniques into your daily life. We'll help you set achievable goals and track your progress.

10. Your Personalized Holistic Stress Management Plan:

Finally, we'll guide you in crafting your personalized holistic stress management plan. You'll have the opportunity to reflect on your unique needs, preferences, and progress, ensuring that your journey towards balance and calm is tailored to you.

By the end of this book, you'll not only have a comprehensive understanding of holistic stress management but also a practical roadmap for implementing these practices into your life. The aim is to empower you to reclaim control over your well-being, find tranquility amidst life's challenges, and create a more relaxed and fulfilling life. Are you ready to explore these holistic approaches together?

Chapter 2: Yoga for Stress Relief

Now, let's delve into the world of yoga and explore how this ancient practice can be a powerful tool for reducing stress and promoting overall well-being.

Principles of Yoga for Stress Reduction:

Yoga is more than just a series of physical postures; it's a holistic system that addresses the mind, body, and spirit. Here are some key principles that underpin yoga's effectiveness in reducing stress:

1. Mind-Body Connection:

- Yoga emphasizes the profound connection between the mind and body. It teaches you to be present in the moment, to listen to your body's signals, and to respond with compassion.

2. Breath Awareness:

- A fundamental aspect of yoga is pranayama, or breath control. It teaches you to regulate your breath, which, in turn, calms the nervous system and reduces stress responses.

3. Mindfulness and Meditation:

- Yoga often incorporates mindfulness and meditation practices. These techniques encourage you to observe your thoughts without judgment, promoting mental clarity and reducing stress-inducing rumination.

4. Physical Postures (Asanas):

- The physical postures of yoga (asanas) promote flexibility, strength, and relaxation. They release physical tension, which can be a reflection of emotional stress.

5. Relaxation and Savasana:

- Each yoga session typically ends with Savasana, a relaxation pose. This practice allows you to surrender to deep relaxation, releasing pent-up stress and tension.

Benefits of Yoga for Stress Reduction:

Now, let's explore the numerous benefits that yoga offers for stress reduction:

1. Stress Hormone Regulation:

- Yoga helps regulate the production of stress hormones like cortisol. By practicing regularly, you can lower these hormone levels, reducing the physiological impact of stress.

2. Relaxation Response:

- Yoga activates the parasympathetic nervous system, known as the "rest and digest" response. This counters the "fight or flight" response, promoting relaxation and reducing stress.

3. Emotional Balance:

- Yoga cultivates emotional stability by promoting self-awareness and self-acceptance. It provides tools to manage emotional reactions and build resilience.

4. Physical Tension Release:

- Through yoga postures, you can release physical tension, which often mirrors emotional stress. Stretching and strengthening the body help relax muscles and alleviate discomfort.

5. Improved Sleep:

- Consistent yoga practice is linked to improved sleep quality. Better sleep not only reduces stress but also enhances overall well-being.

6. Enhanced Mindfulness:

- Yoga fosters mindfulness, enabling you to stay present and engaged in the current moment. This reduces the impact of worries about the past or future.

7. Stress Reduction in Daily Life:

- The mindfulness and relaxation techniques learned in yoga can be applied to everyday situations, helping you navigate daily stressors with greater ease.

8. Increased Resilience:

- Over time, yoga builds mental and emotional resilience, making you better equipped to handle life's challenges without becoming overwhelmed.

Incorporating yoga into your life can be a transformative journey towards stress reduction and holistic well-being. In the upcoming sections of this chapter, we'll delve deeper into the practical aspects of yoga for stress relief. You'll learn specific postures, breathing techniques, and mindfulness practices that you can easily integrate into your daily routine. By the end of this chapter, you'll have the tools to harness the power of yoga and cultivate greater calm and balance in your life. Ready to begin this enlightening exploration of yoga for stress relief?

Basic Yoga Poses for Stress Relief:

1. **Child's Pose (Balasana):**

- Kneel on the floor with your big toes touching and knees apart.
- Sit back on your heels and extend your arms forward, lowering your chest toward the ground.
- Rest your forehead on the floor and breathe deeply. Hold for 30

seconds to 1 minute.

1. **Cat-Cow Pose (Marjaryasana-Bitilasana):**

- Start on your hands and knees in a tabletop position.
- Inhale, arch your back, and lift your head and tailbone (Cow Pose).
- Exhale, round your back, tuck your chin, and tuck your tailbone (Cat Pose).
- Flow between these two poses, syncing your breath with movement for 1-2 minutes.

1. **Downward-Facing Dog (Adho Mukha Svanasana):**

- Begin in a push-up position with your hands shoulder-width apart.
- Push your hips up and back, forming an inverted "V" shape with your body.
- Press your heels toward the ground and lengthen your spine. Hold for 30 seconds to 1 minute.

1. **Standing Forward Bend (Uttanasana):**

- Stand with your feet hip-width apart.
- Exhale and bend forward at your hips, keeping your knees slightly bent.
- Let your upper body hang down, and bring your hands to the floor or grab your elbows.
- Hold for 30 seconds to 1 minute.

Breathing Exercises for Stress Relief:

1. **Deep Belly Breathing:**

- Sit or lie down in a comfortable position.
- Place one hand on your chest and the other on your abdomen.
- Inhale deeply through your nose, expanding your abdomen.
- Exhale slowly through your mouth, feeling your abdomen fall.

- Continue for several minutes, focusing on deep, rhythmic breaths.

1. **4-7-8 Breath:**

- Sit or lie down with your eyes closed.
- Inhale quietly through your nose to a mental count of 4.
- Hold your breath for a count of 7.
- Exhale completely through your mouth to a count of 8.
- Repeat this cycle four times, gradually increasing with practice.

1. **Alternate Nostril Breathing (Nadi Shodhana):**

- Sit in a comfortable position with your spine straight.
- Close your right nostril with your right thumb and inhale through your left nostril.
- Close your left nostril with your right ring finger and release the right nostril.
- Exhale through your right nostril.
- Inhale through your right nostril, close it, and release the left nostril.
- Exhale through your left nostril.
- Repeat for several cycles, focusing on slow and controlled breaths.

Remember that yoga and breathing exercises are most effective when practiced regularly. Start with a few minutes each day and gradually increase your practice duration. Pay attention to your body, and don't push yourself into discomfort. These practices are meant to be calming and nurturing, so honor your own pace and limitations. Over time, you'll find that they become valuable tools for reducing stress and promoting relaxation in your daily life.

Success Story 1: Sarah's Journey to Inner Peace

Sarah was a busy professional juggling a demanding job, family responsibilities, and a chaotic daily schedule. She often felt overwhelmed and struggled with stress-related health issues, including anxiety and insomnia. Searching for a solution, she decided to give yoga a try.

After just a few weeks of regular yoga practice, Sarah noticed a remarkable change. Her anxiety levels reduced, and she found herself better equipped to manage challenging situations at work and home. The mindfulness and deep breathing techniques she learned in yoga class became her go-to tools for staying calm under pressure.

Yoga also improved Sarah's sleep quality. She started experiencing restful nights, waking up feeling refreshed and energized. As a result, her overall health improved, and she was able to engage more fully with her family and work.

Sarah's journey with yoga wasn't just about physical postures; it was a transformation of her entire well-being. She continues to practice yoga regularly, not only for stress relief but also for the sense of inner peace and balance it brings to her life.

Success Story 2: John's Recovery from Trauma

John had experienced a traumatic event that left him with post-traumatic stress disorder (PTSD). His life was marked by anxiety, nightmares, and a constant sense of dread. Traditional therapies had provided some relief, but he was still searching for a more profound healing experience.

Upon the recommendation of a friend, John joined a yoga class specifically designed for individuals dealing with trauma and stress. Initially, it was challenging for him to be in a group setting, but he found comfort in the supportive and non-judgmental environment the class provided.

Through yoga, John learned to reconnect with his body and emotions. The practice of mindfulness and controlled breathing allowed him to confront his fears and anxieties with greater resilience. Over time, he started to experience a sense of calm and safety that had eluded him for years.

Yoga became an integral part of John's healing process. While he acknowledges that recovery from trauma is a journey, he credits yoga with helping him regain control of his life and find relief from the burdens of PTSD. Today, John continues his yoga practice and has even become an advocate for yoga as a complementary therapy for trauma survivors.

These real-life success stories illustrate the transformative power of yoga as a tool for managing stress, promoting mental health, and finding inner peace. While everyone's journey is unique, these stories demonstrate that with dedication and the right support, yoga can be a profound source of relief and healing in the face of life's challenges.

Finding Local Yoga Classes:

1. **Online Research:** Start your search online by looking for yoga studios, wellness centers, or community centers in your area. Many of them have websites or social media profiles where they list class schedules and descriptions.
2. **Yoga Directories:** Websites and apps like YogaFinder, YogaTrail, or Mindbody often provide comprehensive listings of yoga classes and studios in various locations. You can search by location, style, and teacher.
3. **Ask for Recommendations:** Seek recommendations from friends, family, or coworkers who practice yoga. They may have insights into the best local instructors and studios.
4. **Visit Studios:** Take the time to visit local yoga studios or centers in person. Attend a class or two as a drop-in student to get a feel for the atmosphere, teaching style, and community.
5. **Community Centers and Gyms:** Check out your local community centers, gyms, or recreation centers. They often offer yoga classes as part of their fitness programs at affordable rates.
6. **Meetup Groups:** Websites like Meetup.com may have yoga groups in your area. These groups often organize yoga events, classes, or gatherings.
7. **Yoga Festivals and Events:** Keep an eye out for yoga festivals or events happening in your region. These can be a great way to explore different yoga styles and connect with local instructors.

Practicing Yoga at Home:

1. **Create a Dedicated Space:** Designate a specific area in your home

for yoga practice. It doesn't need to be large; even a corner with a yoga mat will suffice.

2. **Choose a Suitable Time:** Establish a regular practice schedule that works for you. Consistency is key, so pick a time when you're least likely to be interrupted.

3. **Online Yoga Classes:** There are numerous online platforms that offer yoga classes and tutorials, ranging from free resources on YouTube to subscription-based services like YogaGlo, Yoga International, or Glo. You can choose classes based on your level and preferred style.

4. **Use Yoga Apps:** There are several yoga apps available for smartphones and tablets that provide guided yoga sessions, from beginner to advanced levels.

5. **Invest in Props:** Consider purchasing basic yoga props like a mat, blocks, and a strap to support your home practice. These props can enhance your experience and help you perform poses safely.

6. **Follow a Routine:** Find a beginner's yoga routine or video that suits your needs. Start with shorter sessions and gradually increase the duration as you become more comfortable.

7. **Stay Consistent:** Consistency is essential for progress in yoga. Aim to practice regularly, even if it's just for a few minutes each day. Set achievable goals to stay motivated.

8. **Seek Online Communities:** Join online yoga communities or forums where you can connect with other practitioners. Sharing your experiences and challenges can help keep you accountable.

9. **Consider Online Classes:** Some yoga studios now offer live-streamed or pre-recorded classes. You can participate from home while still benefiting from the guidance of an instructor.

10. **Mindful Practice:** Remember that yoga is not just about physical postures; it's also about mindfulness and self-awareness. Embrace the mental and emotional benefits of yoga as you practice at home.

Whether you choose to attend local classes or practice at home, the key is to find a routine that resonates with you and supports your stress relief goals. Yoga is a journey of self-discovery and self-care, and it's important to approach it with patience and an open heart.

The Mind-Body Connection in Yoga

In the practice of yoga, the mind-body connection is not merely a concept; it's a fundamental principle that underpins the transformative power of this ancient discipline. Here, we emphasize the profound mind-body connection in yoga practice and how it contributes to stress relief and holistic well-being.

1. **Awareness of Breath:** Yoga places significant emphasis on breath awareness. Through conscious breathing, you connect your mind with the physical act of inhaling and exhaling. This awareness calms the mind, reduces mental chatter, and relaxes the body.

2. **Physical Postures (Asanas):** The practice of yoga postures, or asanas, is a tangible embodiment of the mind-body connection. As you move through poses, you become acutely aware of how your body feels in each moment. This awareness fosters a sense of presence and mindfulness.

3. **Release of Physical Tension:** Many physical postures in yoga are designed to release physical tension and tightness in the body. As you stretch and strengthen muscles, you simultaneously release emotional and mental tension that may be stored in the body.

4. **Integration of Breath and Movement:** In yoga, the synchronization of breath with movement is central. Each asana is accompanied by a specific breath pattern. This connection not only enhances the effectiveness of the pose but also deepens your awareness of the breath-movement relationship.

5. **Mindfulness Meditation:** Yoga often incorporates mindfulness meditation practices. These techniques encourage you to observe your thoughts without judgment. By cultivating this skill, you learn to distance yourself from stress-inducing thoughts and emotions.

Benefits of the Mind-Body Connection in Yoga:

1. **Stress Reduction:** The conscious awareness of breath and the body's

sensations in yoga helps reduce stress responses. You learn to remain calm and composed even in challenging situations.

2. **Emotional Regulation:** Yoga enhances emotional regulation by teaching you to observe and manage emotional reactions. It promotes a sense of emotional balance and resilience.

3. **Physical Relaxation:** The mind-body connection in yoga promotes physical relaxation. You release muscular tension, which often mirrors emotional stress, leading to a deep sense of relaxation.

4. **Enhanced Focus and Concentration:** The practice of mindfulness in yoga improves your ability to focus and concentrate. This heightened awareness can be applied to tasks in daily life, reducing distractions and stress.

5. **Improved Sleep Quality:** The relaxation and mindfulness techniques learned in yoga can lead to improved sleep quality. You're better equipped to quiet a restless mind and experience restorative sleep.

6. **Increased Self-Awareness:** Yoga cultivates self-awareness, allowing you to recognize the sources of stress in your life. This awareness empowers you to make conscious choices to reduce stress.

7. **A Holistic Approach to Well-being:** By integrating the mind and body in yoga practice, you address stress on multiple levels. This holistic approach contributes to overall well-being, promoting balance and harmony.

As you progress in your yoga practice, you'll continually deepen your understanding of the mind-body connection. It's a journey of self-discovery and self-care that has the power to transform how you relate to stress and how you experience life itself. Remember that yoga is not a destination but a lifelong exploration, and the mind-body connection is your guiding light on this path to stress relief and holistic well-being.

Chapter 3: The Power of Meditation

Meditation is a practice that has been revered for centuries for its profound effects on the mind, body, and spirit. In recent years, scientific research has begun to unravel the mechanisms behind meditation and its impact on the brain. Let's delve into the science behind meditation and how it influences our brain and overall well-being.

Understanding Meditation and Its Varieties:

Meditation encompasses a wide range of practices, but they all share a common goal: to quiet the mind and promote a sense of inner peace. Some popular meditation techniques include mindfulness meditation, loving-kindness meditation (Metta), transcendental meditation (TM), and Zen meditation, among others.

The Science Behind Meditation:

1. **Brain Structure Changes:** Numerous studies using neuroimaging techniques like MRI have shown that regular meditation can lead to structural changes in the brain. For example, the hippocampus, which is associated with memory and learning, tends to increase in size in meditators. The amygdala, involved in the processing of emotions, often shows reduced activity.
2. **Enhanced Connectivity:** Meditation appears to enhance connectivity between different regions of the brain. This increased connectivity can foster improved cognitive function, emotional regulation, and overall mental well-being.
3. **Reduction in Stress Response:** Meditation is renowned for its ability to reduce the body's stress response. Through practices like mindfulness meditation, individuals can learn to regulate their body's production of stress hormones like cortisol, leading to decreased stress levels.
4. **Changes in Grey Matter:** Studies have reported increased grey matter density in brain regions associated with attention, memory,

and self-awareness in meditation practitioners. These changes are believed to contribute to improved cognitive function.

5. **Enhanced Focus and Attention:** Regular meditation is associated with better focus and attention. This is evident in studies that show improvements in tasks requiring sustained attention, problem-solving, and decision-making.

6. **Emotional Regulation:** Meditation practices, such as loving-kindness meditation, can lead to greater emotional regulation. This is linked to changes in the prefrontal cortex, which is responsible for emotional processing and control.

7. **Pain Management:** Meditation has been shown to modulate the perception of pain. Studies indicate that meditators can endure pain for longer periods without experiencing the same level of discomfort as non-meditators.

8. **Improved Sleep:** Meditation can positively influence sleep quality by calming the mind and reducing sleep disturbances. It's particularly helpful for individuals with insomnia or sleep-related issues.

9. **Reduction in Symptoms of Anxiety and Depression:** Meditation has been recognized as a complementary approach for managing anxiety and depressive disorders. It helps individuals gain perspective on their thoughts and emotions, reducing the impact of these conditions.

10. **Greater Overall Well-being:** Perhaps most importantly, meditation is associated with an overall sense of well-being and life satisfaction. It fosters a positive outlook on life and greater resilience in the face of adversity.

The Role of Neuroplasticity:

Neuroplasticity, the brain's ability to adapt and reorganize, plays a crucial role in the benefits of meditation. As individuals engage in regular meditation, their brains undergo structural and functional changes that enhance mental and emotional resilience.

The science behind meditation reveals that it is not just a subjective experience; it is a profound process that can lead to tangible changes in the brain, contributing to improved mental and emotional well-being. These findings underscore the importance of integrating meditation into your daily routine as a valuable tool for stress reduction and holistic well-being. In the following sections of this chapter, we will explore various meditation techniques and how to incorporate them into your life to unlock their transformative potential.

1. Mindfulness Meditation:

In this chapter, we'll explore several meditation techniques, each offering unique benefits for stress reduction, emotional well-being, and personal growth. Let's dive into two widely-practiced meditation approaches: Mindfulness Meditation and Loving-Kindness Meditation (Metta).

Mindfulness meditation is perhaps one of the most well-known and widely practiced forms of meditation. It involves paying focused attention to the present moment without judgment. Here's how to practice mindfulness meditation:

- Find a quiet and comfortable space to sit or lie down.
- Close your eyes and take a few deep breaths to center yourself.
- Shift your attention to your breath. Observe the sensation of your breath as it enters and leaves your nostrils or the rise and fall of your abdomen.
- When your mind wanders (as it inevitably will), gently bring your focus back to your breath without self-criticism.
- Notice any thoughts, sensations, or emotions that arise without attachment or judgment. Let them come and go like clouds in the sky.
- Practice for a set amount of time, starting with a few minutes and gradually extending your sessions as you become more comfortable.

Mindfulness meditation enhances self-awareness, reduces stress, and cultivates a sense of presence and clarity.

2. Loving-Kindness Meditation (Metta):

Loving-Kindness Meditation, also known as Metta, is a practice that fosters feelings of love, compassion, and goodwill towards oneself and others. Here's how to practice Loving-Kindness Meditation:

- Find a quiet and comfortable place to sit or lie down.
- Close your eyes and take a few deep breaths to center yourself.
- Begin by directing loving-kindness towards yourself. Silently repeat phrases like, "May I be happy, may I be healthy, may I live with ease."
- Next, extend these wishes to a loved one. Picture them in your mind and repeat the phrases, such as, "May you be happy, may you be healthy, may you live with ease."
- Gradually, broaden your circle of compassion to include acquaintances, difficult people, and eventually all living beings.
- Feel the warmth and goodwill radiating from your heart as you extend these wishes.
- Practice for a set amount of time, starting with a few minutes and increasing the duration over time.

Loving-Kindness Meditation enhances empathy, fosters positive emotions, and promotes a sense of interconnectedness with all beings.

Other Meditation Techniques:

While Mindfulness and Loving-Kindness Meditation are two of the most widely practiced forms, there are numerous other meditation techniques, including:

- **Transcendental Meditation (TM):** Involves silently repeating a mantra to achieve a state of deep rest and relaxation.
- **Zen Meditation (Zazen):** Focuses on seated meditation and observing the breath and thoughts without attachment.
- **Guided Meditation:** Involves listening to a recorded meditation led by an instructor, often focusing on specific themes or goals.
- **Body Scan Meditation:** Involves systematically scanning and relaxing different parts of the body to release tension.

Exploring various meditation techniques allows you to find the approach that resonates most with you and meets your specific needs. Whether you choose mindfulness, loving-kindness, or another form of meditation, regular practice can lead to profound benefits in reducing stress, enhancing emotional well-being, and promoting a greater sense of inner peace and balance.

1. Choose the Location:

Creating a tranquil and dedicated meditation space is essential for a harmonious and effective meditation practice. Here's a step-by-step guide to help you establish your peaceful meditation space.

Select a location in your home or another quiet place where you can meditate without interruptions. It could be a spare room, a corner of your bedroom, or even a cozy nook in your living room. The key is to find a spot where you feel comfortable and can focus.

2. Clear the Clutter:

Before setting up your meditation space, declutter the area. Remove any items that might distract you or create visual clutter. A clean and organized space is conducive to a peaceful mind.

3. Arrange Comfortable Seating:

Choose a comfortable chair, cushion, or meditation bench to sit on during your practice. Ensure that it provides proper support and encourages good posture. If you prefer sitting on the floor, invest in a cushion or mat that suits your needs.

4. Add Symbolic Items:

Consider adding symbolic items that hold personal meaning and enhance the ambiance of your meditation space. This could include:

- **Incense or Candles:** Scented candles or incense can create a calming atmosphere. Use unscented varieties if you're sensitive to smells.
- **Soothing Colors:** Choose soothing and calming colors for your meditation space. Earth tones, pastels, and soft blues or greens are

often recommended.

- **Inspiring Art or Quotes:** Hang artwork or quotes that inspire you and align with your meditation practice. These can serve as visual focal points.

5. Include Natural Elements:

Bringing in elements of nature can enhance the tranquility of your meditation space. Consider adding:

- **Indoor Plants:** Plants not only purify the air but also create a connection to the natural world.
- **Natural Light:** If possible, meditate in a space with natural light. Sunlight can elevate your mood and energy.

6. Set Up a Meditation Altar:

If you like, create a small meditation altar or shrine. This can be a dedicated space for items that hold spiritual or personal significance:

- **A Statue or Image:** Place a statue or image of a spiritual figure or symbol that resonates with you.
- **Candles or Incense:** Add candles, incense, or other offerings to create a sacred atmosphere.
- **Personal Items:** Include personal items like a meaningful crystal, a mala (prayer beads), or a small bowl for offerings.

7. Keep It Clean and Organized:

Regularly clean and tidy your meditation space. A clutter-free environment fosters a sense of peace and serenity. Make it a habit to put away any items that aren't part of your meditation practice.

8. Create a Routine:

Establish a consistent meditation routine in your space. The act of returning to the same space each day can signal to your mind that it's time for meditation.

Consistency reinforces the connection between your meditation space and your practice.

9. Personalize Your Space:

Remember that your meditation space is a reflection of your personal journey. Feel free to personalize it further with items that hold deep meaning to you, whether they're religious or spiritual symbols, family heirlooms, or anything else that brings you peace and joy.

10. Silence and Privacy:

Ensure that your meditation space offers the privacy and quiet you need for your practice. Communicate with family members or housemates about your meditation times, so they can respect your space and practice.

By creating a peaceful meditation space, you provide yourself with a dedicated sanctuary for your practice. This space becomes a haven where you can cultivate inner peace, reduce stress, and deepen your connection with yourself. Whether your meditation space is simple or elaborate, what matters most is that it supports your journey towards greater well-being and mindfulness.

1. Stress Reduction:

A regular meditation practice can be transformative, impacting every aspect of your life. Let's explore the wide-ranging benefits that come with making meditation a consistent part of your daily routine.

- One of the most well-documented benefits of meditation is its ability to reduce stress. Regular meditation helps lower the production of stress hormones like cortisol, leading to a calmer and more relaxed state of mind.

2. Improved Emotional Well-being:

- Meditation enhances emotional regulation by helping you become more aware of your thoughts and emotions. It enables you to respond to challenging situations with greater equanimity and less reactivity.

3. Enhanced Focus and Concentration:

- Meditation cultivates your ability to concentrate and stay present. This heightened focus extends beyond your meditation sessions, improving your productivity and efficiency in daily tasks.

4. Greater Self-Awareness:

- Through meditation, you gain a deeper understanding of yourself. You become more attuned to your inner thoughts, desires, and motivations, leading to greater self-awareness and self-acceptance.

5. Improved Sleep Quality:

- Many people report improved sleep patterns as a result of regular meditation. The relaxation and mindfulness techniques can help quiet a restless mind and promote restorative sleep.

6. Enhanced Relationships:

- Meditation fosters empathy and compassion, leading to more harmonious and meaningful relationships. It helps you become a better listener and cultivates a deeper understanding of others.

7. Pain Management:

- Meditation has been shown to modulate the perception of pain. It can be a valuable tool for individuals dealing with chronic pain, offering relief and reducing the need for pain medication.

8. Lower Blood Pressure:

- Regular meditation has been linked to reduced blood pressure, which can contribute to better cardiovascular health.

9. Increased Resilience:

- Meditation builds mental and emotional resilience, helping you navigate life's challenges with greater ease and adaptability.

10. Sense of Peace and Well-being:

- Ultimately, the consistent practice of meditation leads to a profound sense of inner peace and well-being. It enables you to find contentment and joy in the present moment, regardless of external circumstances.

11. Spiritual Growth:

- For those on a spiritual path, meditation can deepen their connection with their inner selves and the universe. It's a powerful tool for self-transcendence and personal growth.

12. Reduced Anxiety and Depression:

- Meditation has been recognized as a complementary approach for managing anxiety and depressive disorders. It helps individuals gain perspective on their thoughts and emotions, reducing the impact of these conditions.

13. Greater Mindfulness:

- Mindfulness, a quality cultivated through meditation, allows you to experience life with heightened awareness. You become fully engaged in each moment, savoring life's richness.

14. Increased Creativity:

- Meditation can boost your creativity by quieting the inner critic and allowing new ideas and insights to surface.

15. Overall Well-being:

- Regular meditation contributes to your overall well-being, promoting balance and harmony in your life. It helps you align with your true self and live in alignment with your values.

These benefits underscore the value of a regular meditation practice as a tool for stress management, emotional well-being, and personal growth. Whether you're new to meditation or have been practicing for years, the rewards of consistency are attainable and deeply enriching. As you continue on your meditation journey, you'll discover that its benefits extend far beyond the time you spend on the cushion, permeating every aspect of your life.

Before delving deeper into your meditation journey, it's important to address common challenges and misconceptions that may arise. By acknowledging and dispelling these concerns, you can approach meditation with a clear and open mind.

Common Challenges in Meditation:

1. **Restless Mind:** It's common to experience a wandering or restless mind during meditation. Thoughts may arise, and you might find it challenging to maintain focus. This is a normal part of the practice. The key is to gently bring your attention back to your chosen point of focus, such as your breath.
2. **Impatience:** Some beginners may become impatient if they don't experience immediate results. Meditation is a gradual process, and its benefits often unfold over time. Cultivate patience and view your practice as a journey rather than a destination.
3. **Physical Discomfort:** Physical discomfort, such as stiffness or pain, can be a distraction during meditation. Ensure you're in a comfortable posture, use cushions or props if necessary, and remember that discomfort is temporary and part of the process.
4. **Lack of Time:** Many people feel they don't have enough time for meditation. Start with short sessions and gradually increase the duration as you build your practice. Even a few minutes of daily meditation can be beneficial.
5. **Inconsistency:** Maintaining a regular meditation routine can be

challenging due to busy schedules. Overcome this by setting realistic goals and integrating meditation into your daily routine, such as meditating before or after other daily habits.

Common Misconceptions About Meditation:

1. **Meditation is About Clearing the Mind Completely:** Contrary to popular belief, meditation is not about emptying the mind entirely. It's about observing your thoughts without attachment or judgment and cultivating mindfulness.
2. **You Need to Achieve a Specific State:** There is no specific "meditation state" that you must attain. Each meditation session is unique, and your experience may vary. Let go of expectations and embrace the present moment.
3. **It's a Religious Practice:** While meditation is a part of many spiritual traditions, it doesn't require a specific religious belief. It can be approached in a secular, non-religious way as a tool for well-being and self-discovery.
4. **Meditation is Time-Consuming:** You don't need to meditate for hours each day to experience benefits. Even brief, consistent sessions can make a significant difference in your life.
5. **It's Only for "Spiritual" People:** Meditation is for everyone, regardless of their spiritual beliefs or background. It's a practical tool that can benefit individuals from all walks of life.
6. **Meditation is a Quick Fix:** Meditation is not a quick fix for all life's problems. It's a process that requires dedication and patience. While it can offer immediate relief from stress, its long-term benefits often unfold gradually.
7. **You Shouldn't Experience Any Discomfort:** Discomfort, physically or mentally, may arise during meditation. It's an opportunity for self-awareness and growth. If the discomfort becomes overwhelming, it's okay to adjust your posture or take a short break.

Understanding these common challenges and dispelling misconceptions can help you approach meditation with greater confidence and a realistic perspective. Embrace the journey of meditation with an open heart and a willingness to learn from every experience, knowing that its rewards extend far beyond the initial hurdles or doubts.

Chapter 4: Aromatherapy for Stress Reduction

Aromatherapy is a holistic practice that harnesses the therapeutic properties of essential oils to promote physical, mental, and emotional well-being. In this chapter, we will explore the fundamentals of aromatherapy and essential oils, including how they work and their benefits for stress reduction.

Understanding Aromatherapy:

1. What Is Aromatherapy?

Aromatherapy is the art and science of using aromatic plant extracts, known as essential oils, to improve overall health and well-being. These essential oils are derived from various parts of plants, such as flowers, leaves, bark, and roots, and are prized for their potent natural fragrances and therapeutic properties.

2. How Does Aromatherapy Work?

Aromatherapy works through the inhalation of aromatic molecules or the application of diluted essential oils to the skin. When you inhale these molecules, they interact with the olfactory system and the limbic system in the brain, which plays a key role in regulating emotions and stress responses. This interaction can have a profound impact on your mood and emotions.

Understanding Essential Oils:

1. What Are Essential Oils?

Essential oils are highly concentrated, volatile compounds extracted from plants. They contain the plant's natural aroma and are packed with therapeutic properties. Each essential oil has a unique chemical composition and offers specific benefits.

2. Methods of Extraction:

Essential oils are extracted through various methods, including steam distillation, cold pressing, and solvent extraction. The method used depends on the type of plant and the specific compounds to be extracted.

3. Diverse Aromatic Profiles:

Essential oils come in a wide range of scents, from floral and citrusy to earthy and woody. Some common essential oils used in aromatherapy for stress reduction include lavender, chamomile, rose, bergamot, and frankincense, among others.

4. Carrier Oils:

To apply essential oils safely to the skin, they are often diluted with carrier oils like jojoba, coconut, or sweet almond oil. This ensures that the essential oil is gentle on the skin and reduces the risk of irritation.

Benefits of Aromatherapy for Stress Reduction:

1. Stress Relief:

Aromatherapy is known for its calming and stress-reducing effects. Certain essential oils, such as lavender and chamomile, can help relax the mind and body, alleviating stress and anxiety.

2. Improved Sleep:

Many essential oils have sedative properties that can improve sleep quality. Diffusing oils like lavender or cedarwood in the bedroom can promote restful sleep.

3. Mood Enhancement:

Aromatherapy can uplift mood and boost emotional well-being. Citrus oils like bergamot and lemon are often used to enhance mood and increase feelings of positivity.

4. Headache and Muscle Tension Relief:

Essential oils like peppermint and eucalyptus can help alleviate headaches and relieve muscle tension when applied topically in a diluted form.

5. Mindfulness and Relaxation:

Aromatherapy encourages mindfulness and relaxation, making it an excellent complement to meditation and other relaxation techniques.

6. Holistic Healing:

Aromatherapy is a holistic approach to well-being, addressing both physical and emotional aspects of stress. It can be integrated into various self-care practices.

Safety Considerations:

While aromatherapy is generally safe when used as directed, it's essential to consider individual sensitivities and allergies. Some essential oils may not be suitable for certain medical conditions or during pregnancy. Always dilute essential oils and perform a patch test before using them on the skin.

In the following sections of this chapter, we will delve into specific essential oils, application methods, and practical tips for incorporating aromatherapy into your stress management routine. By understanding the fundamentals of aromatherapy and essential oils, you can harness their therapeutic benefits for a calmer, more balanced life.

Specific scents have the remarkable ability to influence mood and induce relaxation. In this section, we'll explore how different essential oils and their scents can impact your emotional well-being and create a sense of calm:

1. Lavender:

- **Mood Influence:** Lavender is renowned for its soothing and calming properties. Its scent is often associated with relaxation and stress relief. Inhaling lavender can reduce anxiety and promote a sense of tranquility.
- **Relaxation Benefits:** Lavender essential oil is particularly effective in

promoting better sleep. Diffusing lavender in your bedroom or adding a few drops to your pillow can help you unwind and enjoy a restful night's sleep.

2. Chamomile:

- **Mood Influence:** Chamomile essential oil has a gentle and comforting aroma. It is known for its ability to reduce irritability, anxiety, and emotional tension. Inhaling chamomile can promote a sense of inner peace.
- **Relaxation Benefits:** Chamomile is excellent for relaxation and stress relief. You can add a few drops to a warm bath or use it in massage oil to unwind after a long day.

3. Bergamot:

- **Mood Influence:** Bergamot essential oil has a bright and uplifting citrus scent. It is known for its mood-enhancing properties and can boost feelings of joy and positivity. Inhaling bergamot can help alleviate mild depression and stress.
- **Relaxation Benefits:** Bergamot is an excellent choice for diffusing in your workspace to create a cheerful and stress-free environment.

4. Rose:

- **Mood Influence:** Rose essential oil has a sweet and floral scent that is associated with love and emotional balance. It can help reduce feelings of sadness, anxiety, and grief, promoting emotional healing.
- **Relaxation Benefits:** Rose essential oil is often used in aromatherapy to soothe the emotions and cultivate a sense of self-love and acceptance. It can be added to bathwater or used in massages to enhance relaxation.

5. Frankincense:

- **Mood Influence:** Frankincense essential oil has a woody and earthy scent that is deeply grounding. It can promote feelings of inner peace, spiritual connection, and mental clarity.
- **Relaxation Benefits:** Frankincense is an excellent choice for meditation and mindfulness practices. Inhaling its aroma can help calm the mind and reduce anxiety.

6. Ylang Ylang:

- **Mood Influence:** Ylang ylang essential oil has a sweet and exotic floral scent. It is known for its ability to reduce feelings of stress and promote a sense of happiness and relaxation.
- **Relaxation Benefits:** Ylang ylang is often used in perfumes and body oils. Adding a few drops to your bath or diffuser can create a luxurious and stress-relieving experience.

7. Peppermint:

- **Mood Influence:** Peppermint essential oil has a refreshing and invigorating scent. It can help improve focus, mental clarity, and alertness, reducing feelings of fatigue and mental stress.
- **Relaxation Benefits:** Peppermint is excellent for reducing tension headaches and muscle soreness. Diluted peppermint oil can be applied topically to ease physical tension.

8. Eucalyptus:

- **Mood Influence:** Eucalyptus essential oil has a crisp and invigorating scent that can clear the mind and promote mental clarity. It is often used to reduce mental fatigue.
- **Relaxation Benefits:** Eucalyptus is commonly used to relieve respiratory congestion. Inhaling its aroma can help you breathe more deeply and relax, especially when dealing with colds or sinus congestion.

9. Sandalwood:

- **Mood Influence:** Sandalwood essential oil has a warm and woody scent that encourages introspection and a sense of inner peace. It can help reduce anxiety and promote emotional balance.
- **Relaxation Benefits:** Sandalwood is often used in meditation and spiritual practices. Inhaling its aroma can create a sacred and peaceful atmosphere.

10. Lemon:

- **Mood Influence:** Lemon essential oil has a bright and uplifting citrus scent that can improve mood and reduce stress. It is known for its energizing and cleansing properties.
- **Relaxation Benefits:** Diffusing lemon essential oil in your home can create a fresh and invigorating ambiance, making it an excellent choice for stress relief.

These essential oils and their scents can be incorporated into your daily life through various methods, including diffusing, topical application, inhalation, and adding them to bathwater. Experiment with different scents to discover which ones resonate with you and provide the most profound relaxation and mood-enhancing benefits. Aromatherapy offers a delightful and effective way to reduce stress and create a harmonious atmosphere in your living space.

Here are a few DIY aromatherapy blend recipes that you can create at home to enhance relaxation and reduce stress. These blends can be used in diffusers, added to massage oils, or applied topically (after proper dilution with a carrier oil). Remember to perform a patch test when using new essential oil blends on your skin to ensure you don't have any adverse reactions.

Relaxation Blend:

This blend combines the soothing scents of lavender and chamomile to promote relaxation and ease stress.

- 4 drops of Lavender essential oil
- 3 drops of Roman Chamomile essential oil
- 2 drops of Bergamot essential oil

Energizing Citrus Blend:

If you're looking for an uplifting and invigorating blend, this citrusy combination is perfect.

- 4 drops of Sweet Orange essential oil
- 3 drops of Lemon essential oil
- 2 drops of Grapefruit essential oil
- 1 drop of Peppermint essential oil

Mood-Enhancing Blend:

This blend combines floral and woody notes to enhance mood and promote emotional balance.

- 3 drops of Ylang Ylang essential oil
- 2 drops of Frankincense essential oil
- 2 drops of Geranium essential oil
- 1 drop of Sandalwood essential oil

Sinus Relief Blend:

If you're dealing with congestion or sinus issues, this blend can help you breathe more easily.

- 3 drops of Eucalyptus essential oil
- 2 drops of Peppermint essential oil
- 2 drops of Tea Tree essential oil
- 1 drop of Lemon essential oil

Bedtime Bliss Blend:

This blend is designed to promote a restful night's sleep and reduce nighttime restlessness.

- 4 drops of Lavender essential oil
- 3 drops of Cedarwood essential oil
- 2 drops of Bergamot essential oil

Stress Buster Blend:

When you need quick stress relief, this blend with grounding and calming oils can be your go-to.

- 3 drops of Lavender essential oil
- 2 drops of Frankincense essential oil
- 2 drops of Bergamot essential oil
- 1 drop of Vetiver essential oil

Calming and Centering Blend:

This blend combines earthy and citrusy notes for a calming and centering effect.

- 3 drops of Patchouli essential oil
- 2 drops of Sweet Orange essential oil
- 2 drops of Bergamot essential oil
- 1 drop of Sandalwood essential oil

Note: When using essential oils topically, always dilute them with a carrier oil like jojoba, coconut, or sweet almond oil to avoid skin irritation. The general guideline is to use a 2-3% dilution, which means adding 6-9 drops of essential oil to 1 ounce (30 ml) of carrier oil. Additionally, if you have any allergies or sensitivities, perform a patch test before using a new blend on your skin.

Feel free to adjust the number of drops in these recipes to suit your personal preferences. Aromatherapy blends are highly customizable, allowing you to create scents that resonate with you and provide the relaxation and stress relief you seek.

Before incorporating essential oils into your stress management routine, it's crucial to understand and follow safety precautions to ensure their safe and effective use. Here are important guidelines to consider:

1. Dilution:

Essential oils are highly concentrated and should not be applied directly to the skin in their undiluted form. Always dilute essential oils with a carrier oil, such as jojoba, coconut, or sweet almond oil, before applying them topically. The typical dilution ratio is 2-3% essential oil to carrier oil.

2. Patch Test:

Perform a patch test before using a new essential oil or blend on your skin. Apply a small diluted amount to a discreet area, such as your forearm. Wait 24 hours to check for any allergic reactions, irritation, or sensitivities.

3. Photosensitivity:

Some essential oils, especially citrus oils like lemon and bergamot, can make your skin more sensitive to sunlight. Avoid sun exposure or tanning beds for at least 12 hours after using these oils topically.

4. Avoid Sensitive Areas:

Exercise caution when applying essential oils near sensitive areas, such as the eyes, ears, nose, and mucous membranes. Keep essential oils away from these areas and dilute properly if applying nearby.

5. Pregnancy and Nursing:

Certain essential oils should be avoided during pregnancy and while breastfeeding. Consult with a qualified healthcare professional or aromatherapist before using essential oils if you are pregnant or nursing.

6. Children and Pets:

Use extra caution when using essential oils around children and pets. Some oils are not safe for them, and others should be used in lower concentrations.

Research safe essential oils for their age and species, and store oils out of their reach.

7. Allergies and Sensitivities:

If you have known allergies or sensitivities to specific plants or substances, exercise caution when using essential oils derived from those plants. Cross-referencing the botanical names of essential oils can help you avoid potential allergens.

8. Internal Use:

Ingesting essential oils should only be done under the guidance of a qualified healthcare professional or aromatherapist. Many essential oils are not safe for internal use and can be toxic if ingested.

9. Storage:

Store essential oils in dark glass bottles in a cool, dark place, away from direct sunlight and heat. Proper storage helps preserve their potency and prevents oxidation.

10. Quality Matters:

Invest in high-quality, pure essential oils from reputable suppliers. Poor-quality oils may contain impurities or synthetic additives that can be harmful.

11. Consult a Professional:

If you have underlying health conditions or are taking medications, consult with a healthcare professional or certified aromatherapist before using essential oils. They can provide personalized guidance based on your specific situation.

12. Use as Directed:

Follow recommended guidelines and instructions for the safe use of essential oils, whether in aromatherapy, massage, or topical application.

13. Sensory Sensitivity:

Be mindful of your own sensory sensitivities and preferences. Essential oils have distinct scents, and some may be too strong or unpleasant for your personal taste.

By adhering to these safety precautions and seeking guidance when needed, you can enjoy the therapeutic benefits of essential oils while minimizing the risk of adverse reactions. Aromatherapy can be a powerful tool for stress reduction and relaxation when used responsibly and with awareness.

Let's explore a few case studies of individuals who have experienced the benefits of aromatherapy in managing stress and enhancing their overall well-being:

Case Study 1: Sarah's Sleep Struggles

Background: Sarah, a 34-year-old marketing manager, had been experiencing chronic sleep disturbances due to work-related stress. She often felt anxious before bedtime, leading to restless nights and fatigue during the day.

Aromatherapy Solution: Sarah decided to try aromatherapy to improve her sleep quality. She created a bedtime blend using lavender and chamomile essential oils. She added a few drops of each oil to her diffuser, which she placed in her bedroom.

Results: After just a few nights of using the aromatherapy blend, Sarah noticed a significant improvement in her sleep. She fell asleep more easily and experienced fewer awakenings during the night. Sarah's daytime fatigue diminished, and her overall mood improved. Aromatherapy became an essential part of her nightly routine, helping her manage stress and achieve restorative sleep.

Case Study 2: Mark's Work-Related Stress

Background: Mark, a 42-year-old accountant, was grappling with work-related stress and anxiety. The demands of his job were taking a toll on his mental well-being, leading to tension headaches and persistent worry.

Aromatherapy Solution: Seeking a natural way to alleviate his stress, Mark began using aromatherapy at work. He created a stress-relief roller blend using lavender, frankincense, and bergamot essential oils diluted in a carrier oil. He applied the blend to his wrists and temples throughout the workday.

Results: Mark found that the aromatherapy blend helped him stay calm and focused during hectic work hours. The soothing scents of lavender and frankincense, combined with the uplifting aroma of bergamot, provided a sense of balance. His tension headaches became less frequent, and he felt better equipped to manage workplace stress. Aromatherapy became a valuable tool in Mark's stress management toolkit.

Case Study 3: Emma's Mindfulness Practice

Background: Emma, a 28-year-old yoga instructor, was passionate about holistic wellness. She wanted to deepen her mindfulness meditation practice and enhance her emotional well-being.

Aromatherapy Solution: Emma incorporated aromatherapy into her mindfulness routine. She used a diffuser to disperse a blend of sandalwood and patchouli essential oils during her meditation sessions. The earthy scents created a serene atmosphere, helping her enter a state of deep mindfulness.

Results: With the addition of aromatherapy, Emma found that her meditation practice became more profound and immersive. The grounding scents of sandalwood and patchouli facilitated a deeper connection with her inner self. Emma experienced reduced stress levels, improved emotional balance, and a greater sense of inner peace through the combination of aromatherapy and meditation.

These case studies illustrate how individuals from various backgrounds and lifestyles have incorporated aromatherapy into their daily routines to manage stress, improve sleep, enhance focus, and promote emotional well-being. Aromatherapy offers a versatile and accessible approach to holistic stress management, providing individuals with effective tools to navigate the challenges of modern life.

Chapter 5: Herbal Remedies and Adaptogens

In this chapter, we'll delve into the fascinating world of herbal remedies and adaptogens, exploring their vital role in stress management and overall well-being. Let's begin by introducing the concept of adaptogens and how they can benefit you.

Understanding Adaptogens:

Adaptogens are a class of botanical substances that have been used in traditional medicine for centuries, particularly in ancient systems like Ayurveda and Traditional Chinese Medicine. These remarkable herbs and roots are known for their unique ability to help the body adapt to stressors, whether they are physical, mental, or environmental in nature.

Key Characteristics of Adaptogens:

1. **Balance and Homeostasis:** Adaptogens work by promoting balance and homeostasis within the body. They help regulate various physiological functions, including the stress response, hormone levels, and immune activity.
2. **Non-Specific Action:** Adaptogens have a non-specific action, meaning they can assist the body in coping with a wide range of stressors rather than targeting a specific issue.
3. **Minimal Side Effects:** Adaptogens are generally considered safe with minimal side effects when used as directed. They differ from some pharmaceuticals that may have more pronounced side effects.
4. **Normalizing Effect:** Adaptogens have a normalizing effect on the body's functions. For instance, they can raise low blood pressure or lower high blood pressure, depending on an individual's needs.

Role of Adaptogens in Stress Management:

Adaptogens play a crucial role in stress management by helping the body adapt to and recover from stress more efficiently. Here's how they work:

1. Stress Response Regulation: Adaptogens can modulate the body's stress response, including the release of stress hormones like cortisol. They help prevent excessive stress-induced hormone fluctuations.

2. Enhanced Energy and Endurance: These botanicals can boost physical and mental stamina, allowing you to better withstand stressors and maintain energy levels throughout the day.

3. Improved Cognitive Function: Adaptogens may enhance cognitive function, including memory, focus, and mental clarity, which can be impaired by chronic stress.

4. Immune Support: They can support the immune system, helping your body fend off illnesses that often result from prolonged stress.

5. Emotional Resilience: Adaptogens may improve emotional resilience, making it easier to manage emotional stressors and maintain a positive outlook.

Common Adaptogenic Herbs:

Several adaptogenic herbs are well-known for their stress-reducing properties. Some of the most popular ones include:

- **Rhodiola Rosea:** Known for its ability to enhance physical and mental performance, Rhodiola is often used to combat fatigue and stress.
- **Ashwagandha:** An Ayurvedic herb, ashwagandha is prized for its stress-reducing and mood-stabilizing effects.
- **Panax Ginseng:** Ginseng is known for increasing energy levels and reducing the effects of stress on the body.
- **Holy Basil (Tulsi):** Holy Basil is revered in Ayurvedic medicine for its ability to promote mental clarity, reduce stress, and support overall well-being.
- **Eleuthero (Siberian Ginseng):** Eleuthero is used to increase endurance and resilience, making it valuable in managing chronic stress.

As we explore herbal remedies and adaptogens further in this chapter, you'll discover how to incorporate these natural stress-fighting allies into your daily routine. Adaptogens offer a holistic and gentle approach to stress management, aligning with the theme of this book's holistic approach to well-being.

Let's explore some of the most well-known and widely used herbs and adaptogens, including ashwagandha and ginseng.

1. Ashwagandha (Withania somnifera):

Background: Ashwagandha, also known as Indian ginseng or winter cherry, is an adaptogenic herb deeply rooted in Ayurvedic medicine. It has a long history of use in traditional Indian healing practices.

Benefits: Ashwagandha is renowned for its ability to reduce stress and anxiety. It helps modulate the body's stress response by regulating cortisol levels. Additionally, it promotes better sleep quality and may improve cognitive function.

Usage: Ashwagandha is available in various forms, including capsules, powders, and tinctures. It can be incorporated into daily routines by adding it to smoothies, tea, or taken as a supplement.

2. Panax Ginseng (Asian Ginseng):

Background: Panax ginseng, often referred to as Asian ginseng or Korean ginseng, is one of the most widely studied adaptogens. It has been used in traditional Chinese medicine for centuries.

Benefits: Panax ginseng is known for its energizing properties and its ability to combat fatigue. It can enhance physical and mental stamina, reduce stress, and support immune function.

Usage: Ginseng supplements are available in various forms, including capsules, extracts, and teas. It's commonly consumed as a daily supplement to enhance overall vitality.

3. Rhodiola Rosea:

Background: Rhodiola rosea, also known as Arctic root or golden root, is native to cold regions of Europe and Asia. It has a history of use in Russian and Scandinavian traditional medicine.

Benefits: Rhodiola is prized for its ability to increase resilience to physical and emotional stress. It can improve mental clarity, boost energy, and reduce fatigue.

Usage: Rhodiola supplements are available in various forms. It's often taken as a daily supplement, especially during times of increased stress or fatigue.

4. Holy Basil (Tulsi):

Background: Holy Basil, or Tulsi, is considered a sacred herb in India and is known for its healing properties. It has been used in Ayurveda for thousands of years.

Benefits: Holy Basil is valued for its calming and stress-reducing effects. It can help lower cortisol levels, reduce anxiety, and promote mental clarity. Additionally, it has antioxidant and anti-inflammatory properties.

Usage: Holy Basil is commonly consumed as a tea or taken in supplement form. It can be enjoyed daily to support overall well-being.

5. Eleuthero (Siberian Ginseng):

Background: Eleuthero, also known as Siberian ginseng, is native to Russia and Asia. It has been used in traditional Chinese medicine as an adaptogen.

Benefits: Eleuthero is known for increasing endurance and resilience. It can enhance physical performance, reduce fatigue, and support the immune system.

Usage: Eleuthero is available in various forms, including capsules, tinctures, and teas. It is often used by athletes and individuals seeking to improve stamina.

6. Schisandra Chinensis:

Background: Schisandra chinensis is a berry-bearing vine native to China and Russia. It has a long history of use in traditional Chinese medicine.

Benefits: Schisandra is considered an adaptogen due to its ability to enhance resistance to stress. It may improve mental clarity, reduce fatigue, and support liver function.

Usage: Schisandra is available in supplement form, and its berries can be made into teas or extracts. It is often used to enhance mental focus and energy.

These herbs and adaptogens offer a natural and holistic approach to stress management and overall well-being. They can be integrated into your daily routine to support your body's ability to adapt to stress, enhance resilience, and promote a state of balance and vitality. Whether you choose to incorporate them as supplements, teas, or other forms, these natural remedies can be valuable allies on your journey toward a stress-free and balanced life.

Here are some herbal tea and tincture recipes that can help combat stress and promote relaxation. These recipes use a combination of herbs known for their calming and stress-reducing properties. Remember to consult with a healthcare professional if you have any medical conditions or are taking medications, as some herbs may interact with certain medications.

Calming Herbal Tea:

This soothing herbal tea blend combines several herbs known for their stress-relieving properties.

Ingredients:

- 1 teaspoon of dried lavender flowers
- 1 teaspoon of dried chamomile flowers
- 1 teaspoon of dried lemon balm leaves
- 1 teaspoon of dried passionflower leaves
- 1 cup of boiling water

Instructions:

1. Place the dried herbs in a teapot or a heatproof container.
2. Pour the boiling water over the herbs.

3. Cover and steep for 5-10 minutes.
4. Strain the tea into a cup and enjoy. You can add honey or a slice of lemon for extra flavor.

Stress-Relief Tincture:

A tincture is a concentrated liquid extract of herbs that can be taken in small doses to combat stress. This tincture combines herbs with adaptogenic and calming properties.

Ingredients:

- 1 part ashwagandha root
- 1 part rhodiola root
- 1 part lemon balm leaves
- 1 part passionflower leaves
- 80-proof vodka or brandy

Instructions:

1. Combine equal parts of the dried herbs in a glass jar.
2. Pour enough alcohol (vodka or brandy) to cover the herbs completely. Ensure the alcohol covers the herbs by at least an inch.
3. Seal the jar tightly and shake it vigorously.
4. Store the jar in a cool, dark place for about 4-6 weeks, shaking it daily.
5. After the steeping period, strain the tincture through a fine mesh strainer or cheesecloth into a clean, dark glass dropper bottle.
6. Take 1-2 dropperfuls (about 20-40 drops) in a small amount of water or tea, up to three times a day when needed for stress relief.

Chamomile and Lavender Relaxation Tea:

This simple tea combines two classic calming herbs, chamomile and lavender, for a soothing and relaxing drink.

Ingredients:

- 1 teaspoon of dried chamomile flowers
- 1 teaspoon of dried lavender flowers
- 1 cup of boiling water

Instructions:

1. Place the dried chamomile and lavender flowers in a teapot or cup.
2. Pour the boiling water over the herbs.
3. Cover and steep for 5-10 minutes.
4. Strain the tea into a cup and enjoy. You can add a touch of honey for sweetness if desired.

Passionflower Sleep Tincture:

This tincture combines passionflower, known for its sedative properties, to help promote restful sleep.

Ingredients:

- 1 part dried passionflower leaves
- 80-proof vodka or brandy

Instructions:

1. Place the dried passionflower leaves in a glass jar.
2. Pour enough alcohol (vodka or brandy) to cover the leaves completely.
3. Seal the jar tightly and shake it vigorously.
4. Store the jar in a cool, dark place for about 4-6 weeks, shaking it daily.
5. After the steeping period, strain the tincture through a fine mesh strainer or cheesecloth into a clean, dark glass dropper bottle.
6. Take 1-2 dropperfuls (about 20-40 drops) in a small amount of water about 30 minutes before bedtime to promote restful sleep.

These herbal tea and tincture recipes can be a valuable addition to your stress management toolkit. Enjoy them as part of your daily self-care routine to help combat stress, relax, and promote a sense of calm and well-being.

As you explore the world of herbal remedies and adaptogens for stress management, it's essential to understand the importance of consulting with an herbalist or healthcare professional. While herbs can be powerful allies in your quest for well-being, their use should be guided by expert knowledge and tailored to your individual needs. Here's why consulting with a qualified professional is crucial:

1. Safety and Individualization:

- An herbalist or healthcare professional can assess your specific health history, current medications, and any underlying medical conditions to ensure that the herbal remedies and adaptogens you use are safe and appropriate for you.

2. Correct Dosage and Formulation:

- Herbal remedies can be administered in various forms, including teas, tinctures, capsules, and salves. An expert can recommend the most effective and convenient form for your needs and provide precise dosing instructions.

3. Herb-Drug Interactions:

- Some herbs can interact with prescription medications, potentially leading to adverse effects. A healthcare professional can identify potential interactions and recommend suitable alternatives or adjustments to your treatment plan.

4. Monitoring and Adjustments:

- Regular check-ins with an herbalist or healthcare provider allow for monitoring of your progress and any potential side effects.

Adjustments to your herbal regimen can be made as needed to ensure the best results.

5. Allergies and Sensitivities:

- If you have allergies or sensitivities to specific herbs or plants, an herbalist can help you identify safe alternatives and avoid potential allergic reactions.

6. Comprehensive Knowledge:

- Herbalists and healthcare professionals possess in-depth knowledge of herbs, including their traditional uses, current research, and best practices for preparation and administration.

7. Quality Control:

- Experts can recommend reputable sources for herbal products and ensure that you are using high-quality, contaminant-free herbs.

8. Holistic Assessment:

- Herbalists often take a holistic approach, considering not only the physical aspects of health but also emotional, mental, and lifestyle factors. This comprehensive assessment can lead to a more effective herbal treatment plan.

9. Personalized Guidance:

- Everyone's body and health needs are unique. An herbalist can customize herbal remedies and adaptogen recommendations based on your individual constitution and goals.

10. Maximizing Benefits:

- An herbalist can guide you in creating a well-rounded approach to stress management, incorporating herbs, nutrition, lifestyle changes, and other wellness practices to maximize the benefits of your herbal regimen.

11. Ethical and Sustainable Sourcing:

- Herbalists often prioritize ethical and sustainable sourcing of herbs, supporting environmentally responsible practices and fair trade.

While herbs and adaptogens can be valuable tools for stress management and overall well-being, their safe and effective use is best achieved under the guidance of a qualified herbalist or healthcare professional. Their expertise ensures that you receive personalized and evidence-based recommendations tailored to your specific needs, ultimately leading to the best possible outcomes in your journey toward holistic stress management and improved health.

As you explore herbal remedies and adaptogens for stress management, it's crucial to be aware of potential side effects and contraindications. While many herbs are safe and well-tolerated, they can have effects on the body, and interactions with certain medical conditions or medications may occur. Here's an overview of common side effects and contraindications to keep in mind:

Potential Side Effects of Herbal Remedies:

1. **Allergic Reactions:** Some individuals may be allergic to specific herbs or botanicals. Allergic reactions can range from mild skin irritations to severe reactions like anaphylaxis. It's essential to be cautious if you have known allergies.
2. **Gastrointestinal Disturbances:** Some herbs, especially when taken in high doses, can cause gastrointestinal issues such as nausea, diarrhea, or stomach cramps.
3. **Interactions with Medications:** Certain herbs can interact with prescription and over-the-counter medications, affecting their efficacy or causing adverse effects. Always consult with a healthcare professional if you are taking medications.
4. **Blood Pressure:** Herbs like licorice and ginseng can impact blood

pressure. Individuals with hypertension or low blood pressure should exercise caution when using these herbs.

5. **Hormonal Effects:** Some herbs, such as licorice and fenugreek, can influence hormone levels. Pregnant and breastfeeding individuals, as well as those with hormone-sensitive conditions, should use these herbs under the guidance of a healthcare provider.

6. **Liver Health:** Herbs like kava and comfrey have been associated with liver toxicity. If you have liver conditions or are taking medications that affect the liver, avoid or use these herbs with extreme caution.

7. **Blood Sugar:** Certain herbs, including fenugreek and cinnamon, can affect blood sugar levels. People with diabetes should monitor their blood sugar closely when using these herbs.

Common Contraindications:

1. **Pregnancy and Breastfeeding:** Many herbs have not been extensively studied in pregnant or breastfeeding individuals. Some herbs can stimulate uterine contractions or affect breast milk production, so it's best to consult a healthcare provider before using any herbal remedies during these times.

2. **Children and Infants:** The safety of herbs for children and infants varies widely, and not all herbs are suitable for young age groups. Always consult with a pediatrician or qualified herbalist before giving herbs to children.

3. **Medical Conditions:** People with specific medical conditions, such as kidney disease, liver disease, heart conditions, or autoimmune disorders, should use herbs cautiously and under the guidance of a healthcare provider.

4. **Surgery:** Some herbs can interfere with anesthesia or blood clotting, potentially affecting surgical outcomes. Inform your surgeon about any herbal supplements you are taking if you are scheduled for surgery.

5. **Allergies:** If you have known allergies to certain plants or botanicals, be cautious when using herbs derived from these sources.

6. **Drug Interactions:** Always consult with a healthcare professional

before using herbs if you are taking prescription medications, as interactions can occur.

Safe and Informed Use of Herbal Remedies:

- If you're considering using herbs or adaptogens for stress management, consult with a qualified herbalist or healthcare provider who can assess your individual health history, needs, and potential risks.
- Start with low doses and monitor your body's response to herbal remedies. If you experience any adverse effects, discontinue use and seek medical advice.
- Use high-quality, reputable sources for herbal products to ensure purity and potency.
- Keep your healthcare provider informed about any herbal remedies you are using, especially if you are undergoing medical treatment.
- Remember that individual responses to herbs can vary, and what works well for one person may not have the same effect on another. Personalized guidance is essential for safe and effective herbal use.

By staying informed and seeking guidance when needed, you can harness the potential benefits of herbal remedies and adaptogens for stress management while minimizing the risk of adverse effects.

Chapter 6: Holistic Nutrition for Stress Resilience

In this chapter, we'll explore the powerful connection between diet and stress. While stress is often seen as a psychological or emotional phenomenon, what you eat can significantly impact your ability to manage stress and enhance your overall resilience. Let's emphasize the link between diet and stress:

The Gut-Brain Connection:

One of the key factors highlighting the link between diet and stress is the gut-brain connection. Your gastrointestinal tract, often referred to as the "second brain," houses a complex network of neurons and is deeply intertwined with your central nervous system. This connection allows your gut to communicate with your brain and vice versa.

How Diet Affects Stress:

1. **Nutrient Intake:** Consuming a balanced diet rich in essential nutrients such as vitamins, minerals, and antioxidants provides your body and brain with the necessary building blocks for optimal function. These nutrients play a vital role in regulating mood, neurotransmitter production, and overall brain health.
2. **Inflammation:** Chronic inflammation, often driven by poor dietary choices, is associated with stress and various mental health disorders. An anti-inflammatory diet can help reduce inflammation and promote emotional well-being.
3. **Blood Sugar Regulation:** The foods you eat directly affect your blood sugar levels. Consuming a diet high in refined sugars and carbohydrates can lead to blood sugar spikes and crashes, which can contribute to mood swings and increased stress.
4. **Gut Microbiome:** Your gut is home to trillions of microorganisms that play a crucial role in digestion, immune function, and even mood regulation. A diet rich in fiber, prebiotics, and probiotics can support a healthy gut microbiome, positively impacting mental health.

5. **Stress Hormones:** Certain foods and beverages, such as caffeine and sugary snacks, can stimulate the release of stress hormones like cortisol. Managing your consumption of these substances can help regulate stress responses.

The Role of Mindful Eating:

In addition to the nutritional aspect of diet, how you eat is equally important. Practicing mindful eating involves paying attention to the sensory experience of food, savoring each bite, and eating without distractions. This approach can help reduce stress by promoting a healthier relationship with food and a greater awareness of your body's hunger and fullness cues.

Creating a Stress-Resilient Diet:

- **Whole Foods:** Emphasize whole, unprocessed foods such as fruits, vegetables, whole grains, lean proteins, and healthy fats in your diet. These foods provide essential nutrients and support overall health.
- **Antioxidants:** Consume foods rich in antioxidants, such as berries, leafy greens, and nuts. Antioxidants combat oxidative stress and inflammation in the body.
- **Omega-3 Fatty Acids:** Incorporate sources of omega-3 fatty acids, like fatty fish (salmon, mackerel), flaxseeds, and walnuts, which have been linked to improved mood and reduced stress.
- **Probiotics:** Include probiotic-rich foods like yogurt, kefir, sauerkraut, and kimchi to support a healthy gut microbiome.
- **Balanced Meals:** Aim for balanced meals that include a combination of carbohydrates, protein, and healthy fats to stabilize blood sugar levels.
- **Hydration:** Stay adequately hydrated by drinking water throughout the day. Dehydration can exacerbate stress and fatigue.
- **Moderation:** While it's essential to prioritize nutrient-dense foods, there's room for occasional treats and indulgences. Balance is key.

By understanding the link between diet and stress and making informed dietary choices, you can cultivate a resilient body and mind that are better equipped to handle life's challenges. In the following sections of this chapter, we will delve deeper into specific dietary strategies, meal planning, and mindful eating practices to support your journey towards stress resilience through nutrition.

Understanding the impact of specific foods on stress is crucial for making informed dietary choices. Some foods can exacerbate stress, while others can help alleviate it. Let's explore both categories:

Foods that can exacerbate stress:

1. **Processed Foods:** Highly processed foods, including fast food, sugary snacks, and many packaged convenience foods, are often high in refined sugars, unhealthy fats, and additives. These can lead to blood sugar spikes and crashes, contributing to mood swings and increased stress.
2. **Caffeine:** While some people tolerate caffeine well, excessive consumption of coffee, energy drinks, and certain teas can lead to increased heart rate, anxiety, and disrupted sleep patterns, all of which can exacerbate stress.
3. **Alcohol:** Alcohol is a depressant that can initially provide a sense of relaxation. However, excessive alcohol consumption can disrupt sleep, dehydrate the body, and contribute to feelings of anxiety and depression.
4. **High Sugar Foods:** Foods and beverages with high sugar content can lead to rapid fluctuations in blood sugar levels, resulting in irritability, fatigue, and cravings, all of which can intensify stress.
5. **Salty Foods:** Excessive salt intake can contribute to high blood pressure and water retention, potentially increasing feelings of stress and discomfort.
6. **Trans Fats:** Trans fats, often found in fried and processed foods, can promote inflammation in the body, which has been linked to increased stress and mental health issues.

Foods that can help alleviate stress:

1. **Complex Carbohydrates:** Whole grains like oats, brown rice, and quinoa provide a steady release of energy and support stable blood sugar levels, promoting a more balanced mood.

2. **Leafy Greens:** Vegetables like spinach, kale, and Swiss chard are rich in folate, which may help regulate mood and reduce feelings of stress and anxiety.

3. **Berries:** Berries such as blueberries, strawberries, and raspberries are high in antioxidants, which can combat oxidative stress and inflammation in the body.

4. **Fatty Fish:** Salmon, mackerel, and trout are excellent sources of omega-3 fatty acids, which have been associated with improved mood and reduced stress.

5. **Protein:** Lean sources of protein like poultry, lean beef, tofu, and legumes contain amino acids that support the production of neurotransmitters like serotonin, which can help regulate mood.

6. **Nuts and Seeds:** Almonds, walnuts, and flaxseeds are rich in nutrients like magnesium, which may help reduce stress and anxiety.

7. **Fermented Foods:** Probiotic-rich foods like yogurt, kefir, sauerkraut, and kimchi support a healthy gut microbiome, which is linked to improved mental well-being.

8. **Herbal Teas:** Certain herbal teas, such as chamomile, lavender, and valerian root, have calming properties and can help alleviate stress and promote relaxation.

9. **Dark Chocolate:** In moderation, dark chocolate with a high cocoa content (70% or higher) contains antioxidants and may promote feelings of well-being and relaxation.

10. **Water:** Staying hydrated is essential for overall well-being. Dehydration can lead to increased stress and fatigue.

By making thoughtful choices and incorporating stress-alleviating foods into your diet while reducing or moderating stress-exacerbating foods, you can create a nutritional foundation that supports your body's ability to manage stress and maintain emotional balance. In the following sections, we will delve deeper into meal planning, mindful eating, and specific dietary strategies to enhance your stress resilience through nutrition.

Meal planning is a valuable tool for stress reduction. By thoughtfully organizing your meals and snacks, you can ensure that your diet supports your body's ability to manage stress effectively. Here are some meal planning tips to help you reduce stress:

1. Prioritize Nutrient-Dense Foods:

- Base your meals on whole, nutrient-dense foods such as fruits, vegetables, whole grains, lean proteins, and healthy fats. These foods provide essential vitamins, minerals, and antioxidants that support overall health and mood regulation.

2. Balanced Meals:

- Create balanced meals that include a combination of carbohydrates, protein, and healthy fats. This balance helps stabilize blood sugar levels and provides sustained energy throughout the day.

3. Frequent Meals and Snacks:

- Aim to eat regularly throughout the day to prevent blood sugar fluctuations. Small, balanced meals and snacks can help maintain stable energy levels and reduce feelings of irritability and stress.

4. Fiber-Rich Foods:

- Include fiber-rich foods like whole grains, legumes, and vegetables in your meals. Fiber promotes satiety and supports digestive health, both of which can contribute to stress reduction.

5. Omega-3 Fatty Acids:

- Incorporate sources of omega-3 fatty acids, such as fatty fish (salmon, mackerel), flaxseeds, and walnuts, into your diet. These fats have been linked to improved mood and reduced stress.

6. Mindful Eating:

- Practice mindful eating by paying full attention to your meal. Savor each bite, eat slowly, and minimize distractions. This approach can help you connect with your body's hunger and fullness cues and reduce overeating due to stress.

7. Limit Caffeine and Alcohol:

- Be mindful of your caffeine and alcohol consumption, especially if you are sensitive to these substances. Consider reducing or eliminating them from your diet, particularly in the afternoon and evening, to support better sleep and reduced stress.

8. Hydration:

- Stay adequately hydrated by drinking water throughout the day. Dehydration can exacerbate stress and fatigue.

9. Plan Ahead:

- Set aside time for meal planning and preparation. Create a weekly meal plan that includes a variety of nutritious foods and recipes. Having a plan in place reduces the temptation to make unhealthy food choices when stressed or pressed for time.

10. Batch Cooking:

- Consider batch cooking on the weekends or when you have extra time. Prepare larger quantities of healthy meals and store them for future use. This practice can save time and ensure that you have nutritious options readily available, reducing the temptation to resort to fast food or processed snacks during busy periods.

11. Portable Snacks:

- Keep healthy snacks on hand, especially when you're on the go. Nuts, seeds, fresh fruit, yogurt, and whole-grain crackers are portable options that can help stabilize blood sugar levels and prevent stress-induced hunger.

12. Experiment and Enjoy:

- Explore new recipes and culinary experiences. Cooking and sharing meals with loved ones can be a source of joy and relaxation, counteracting stress.

13. Seek Support:

- If you're unsure about meal planning or have specific dietary concerns, consider working with a registered dietitian or nutritionist. They can provide personalized guidance and support.

By implementing these meal planning tips, you can create a nourishing and stress-reducing dietary routine. Remember that a holistic approach to nutrition not only supports your physical health but also contributes to emotional well-being and resilience in the face of life's challenges.

Hydration and adequate nutrition play vital roles in stress management. They are often underestimated factors that can significantly impact your ability to cope with stress effectively. Let's explore their roles in more detail:

The Role of Hydration:

1. **Cognitive Function:** Dehydration can impair cognitive function, leading to difficulty concentrating, making decisions, and solving problems. When you're adequately hydrated, your brain functions optimally, helping you manage stress more effectively.
2. **Emotional Well-being:** Even mild dehydration can affect mood. It may lead to increased feelings of anxiety, irritability, and stress.

Staying hydrated can help stabilize your emotional state.

3. **Physical Stress:** Dehydration can place additional stress on your body, as it needs to work harder to maintain normal functions. This added physiological stress can exacerbate the effects of psychological stress.

4. **Sleep Quality:** Dehydration can disrupt sleep patterns, leading to poor sleep quality. A well-hydrated body is more likely to experience restful sleep, which is essential for stress recovery.

The Role of Adequate Nutrition:

1. **Energy Balance:** Proper nutrition ensures that your body receives the energy it needs to function efficiently. Imbalances in energy intake and expenditure can lead to fatigue, which can increase susceptibility to stress.

2. **Nutrient Support:** Essential nutrients, including vitamins, minerals, and antioxidants, play crucial roles in maintaining physical and mental health. These nutrients support processes that regulate mood and stress responses.

3. **Stress Hormones:** Balanced nutrition helps regulate the production of stress hormones like cortisol. When your body is well-nourished, it can better manage and recover from the physiological effects of stress.

4. **Inflammation:** A diet rich in anti-inflammatory foods, such as fruits, vegetables, and omega-3 fatty acids, can reduce inflammation in the body. Chronic inflammation is linked to increased stress and mental health issues.

5. **Gut Health:** Proper nutrition supports a healthy gut microbiome, which is closely connected to mood regulation and stress. A balanced diet with fiber-rich foods, prebiotics, and probiotics fosters a resilient gut-brain axis.

6. **Blood Sugar Regulation:** Consuming balanced meals and snacks that include complex carbohydrates, protein, and healthy fats helps stabilize blood sugar levels. Blood sugar imbalances can contribute to mood swings and increased stress.

7. **Hydration:** Adequate fluid intake is essential for overall health, and

it can help your body better cope with stress. Dehydration can exacerbate stress symptoms.

Practical Tips for Hydration and Adequate Nutrition in Stress Management:

1. **Drink Water Regularly:** Aim to drink water throughout the day, even when you're not feeling thirsty. Carry a reusable water bottle to remind yourself to stay hydrated.
2. **Balanced Meals:** Plan meals that include a variety of nutrient-dense foods. Aim for a combination of carbohydrates, lean protein, and healthy fats in each meal.
3. **Healthy Snacking:** Choose healthy snacks like fresh fruit, nuts, yogurt, or whole-grain crackers to maintain stable energy levels throughout the day.
4. **Mindful Eating:** Practice mindful eating to enhance your awareness of hunger and fullness cues. Avoid eating in front of screens or when distracted.
5. **Reduce Processed Foods:** Minimize processed foods, sugary snacks, and excessive caffeine intake, as these can contribute to stress and energy fluctuations.
6. **Incorporate Omega-3s:** Include sources of omega-3 fatty acids, such as fatty fish, flaxseeds, and walnuts, in your diet to support brain health and mood regulation.
7. **Variety of Vegetables:** Consume a variety of colorful vegetables to ensure a broad spectrum of vitamins and antioxidants.
8. **Probiotic Foods:** Include fermented foods like yogurt, kefir, and kimchi to promote a healthy gut microbiome.
9. **Consult a Professional:** If you have specific dietary concerns or health conditions, consider consulting with a registered dietitian or healthcare provider for personalized guidance.

Incorporating hydration and proper nutrition into your daily routine can significantly enhance your stress resilience, mental well-being, and overall quality of life. These foundational elements are essential for maintaining a balanced and healthy body and mind.

Here are some holistic recipes and meal ideas that can help support stress management through nutrition:

Breakfast Ideas:

1. **Oatmeal with Berries and Nuts:**

   - Cook oats with water or your choice of milk.
   - Top with fresh berries, sliced almonds or walnuts, and a drizzle of honey or maple syrup.

1. **Greek Yogurt Parfait:**

   - Layer Greek yogurt with granola, sliced bananas, and a sprinkle of chia seeds.
   - Add a drizzle of honey or a dash of cinnamon for extra flavor.

1. **Avocado Toast:**

   - Toast whole-grain bread and spread ripe avocado on top.
   - Sprinkle with red pepper flakes, a poached egg, and a pinch of salt and pepper.

Lunch Ideas:

1. **Quinoa Salad with Chickpeas:**

   - Combine cooked quinoa with chickpeas, diced cucumber, cherry tomatoes, red onion, and fresh parsley.
   - Dress with olive oil, lemon juice, and a touch of garlic. Add feta cheese if desired.

1. **Mediterranean Wrap:**

- Fill a whole-grain wrap with hummus, roasted red peppers, sliced cucumber, olives, and baby spinach.
- Roll it up and enjoy a flavorful and nutritious lunch.

1. **Veggie and Lentil Soup:**

- Prepare a hearty vegetable and lentil soup with carrots, celery, onion, spinach, and red lentils.
- Season with herbs and spices like thyme, cumin, and paprika.

Dinner Ideas:

1. **Baked Salmon with Quinoa and Asparagus:**

- Season salmon fillets with lemon juice, garlic, and dill.
- Bake until cooked through and serve with cooked quinoa and roasted asparagus.

1. **Stir-Fried Tofu and Vegetables:**

- Stir-fry tofu cubes with a variety of colorful vegetables (bell peppers, broccoli, snow peas) in a light ginger and soy sauce.
- Serve over brown rice or cauliflower rice.

1. **Chickpea and Spinach Curry:**

- Create a flavorful chickpea and spinach curry with onions, tomatoes, garlic, and a blend of spices like turmeric, cumin, and coriander.
- Serve over brown rice or with whole-grain naan bread.

Snack Ideas:

1. **Trail Mix:**
   - Mix together unsalted nuts (almonds, walnuts), dried fruits (apricots, cranberries), and a handful of dark chocolate chips for a satisfying and energizing snack.

2. **Apple Slices with Nut Butter:**
    ◦ Slice apples and dip them in almond or peanut butter for a delicious and nutritious snack.
3. **Greek Yogurt with Berries:**
    ◦ Top a bowl of Greek yogurt with fresh or frozen berries and a drizzle of honey for a quick and filling snack.

These holistic recipes and meal ideas prioritize whole, nutrient-dense foods that can support your overall well-being and stress management. Remember to tailor them to your preferences and dietary needs and enjoy them mindfully to fully benefit from their stress-reducing potential.

Chapter 7: Mindful Movement and Tai Chi

In this chapter, we will explore Tai Chi as a form of mindful movement—a practice that combines physical exercise, meditation, and deep relaxation to promote holistic well-being. Let's begin by introducing Tai Chi:

The Essence of Tai Chi:

Tai Chi, often referred to as "Tai Chi Chuan" or simply "Tai Chi," is an ancient Chinese martial art that has evolved into a graceful and meditative form of exercise. It is characterized by slow, flowing movements and a focus on mindfulness and breath control. Tai Chi is deeply rooted in traditional Chinese philosophy and principles of balance, harmony, and the flow of vital energy, or "Qi" (pronounced "chee").

Key Elements of Tai Chi:

1. **Mindful Movement:** Tai Chi emphasizes deliberate, precise movements that are performed with full awareness. Practitioners focus their attention on the present moment, cultivating a sense of mindfulness.
2. **Breath Awareness:** Proper breathing techniques are integral to Tai Chi. Practitioners synchronize their breath with each movement, promoting relaxation, mental clarity, and enhanced energy flow.
3. **Balance and Posture:** Tai Chi movements are designed to improve balance, posture, and alignment. The practice helps develop a strong and stable foundation for both physical and mental well-being.
4. **Flow and Continuity:** Tai Chi forms, or sequences of movements, are performed in a continuous, flowing manner. The practice encourages a smooth transition between postures, fostering a sense of harmony and unity.
5. **Stress Reduction:** Tai Chi is renowned for its stress-reduction benefits. Its gentle, slow-paced nature calms the nervous system and reduces the production of stress hormones.
6. **Physical Benefits:** While Tai Chi is gentle and low-impact, it offers

numerous physical benefits, including improved flexibility, muscle strength, and joint mobility.

7. **Holistic Wellness:** Tai Chi is considered a holistic practice that promotes the integration of body, mind, and spirit. It can enhance overall well-being, resilience, and inner peace.

The Philosophy of Tai Chi:

Tai Chi is deeply rooted in Daoist philosophy, which emphasizes living in harmony with the natural flow of life and energy. It encourages the cultivation of balance, moderation, and a deep sense of inner calm. The practice of Tai Chi aligns with these principles, allowing individuals to connect with their inner selves and the world around them.

Tai Chi as a Holistic Stress Management Tool:

Tai Chi's gentle and mindful approach makes it an ideal tool for stress management. Regular practice can:

- **Reduce Stress:** Tai Chi's meditative nature helps reduce the physical and psychological effects of stress, promoting relaxation and emotional well-being.
- **Enhance Mindfulness:** Practicing Tai Chi cultivates mindfulness, improving your ability to stay present, reduce mental chatter, and develop a greater sense of self-awareness.
- **Improve Resilience:** By enhancing physical and mental balance, Tai Chi can improve your ability to adapt to life's challenges and bounce back from stressors.
- **Promote Relaxation:** The slow and deliberate movements of Tai Chi induce a state of relaxation, reducing muscle tension and calming the mind.

In the upcoming sections of this chapter, we will delve deeper into the principles and techniques of Tai Chi, explore its health benefits, and provide guidance on how to incorporate this mindful movement practice into your daily life as a powerful tool for stress management and holistic well-being.

Principles and Benefits of Tai Chi for Stress Relief

Tai Chi, with its graceful, flowing movements and emphasis on mindfulness, offers a unique and effective approach to stress relief. It is grounded in ancient Chinese philosophy and principles that promote harmony and balance in both body and mind. Let's delve into the key principles and the myriad benefits of Tai Chi for stress relief:

Principles of Tai Chi:

1. **Mindful Awareness:** Tai Chi encourages practitioners to be fully present in the moment. Each movement is performed with deliberate attention, fostering mindfulness and a deep connection to the body's sensations.
2. **Balanced Energy (Qi):** In traditional Chinese philosophy, Qi is the vital energy that flows through the body. Tai Chi aims to balance the flow of Qi, promoting physical and emotional harmony.
3. **Flowing Movements:** Tai Chi consists of a series of slow, continuous movements that are seamlessly linked. This flowing quality reflects the principle of continuous change and adaptability.
4. **Yin and Yang:** Tai Chi embodies the concept of Yin and Yang, the complementary forces of nature. It seeks to balance these opposing forces within the body and mind, creating equilibrium.

Benefits of Tai Chi for Stress Relief:

1. **Stress Reduction:** Tai Chi's slow, deliberate movements and emphasis on breath control induce a state of relaxation, reducing the production of stress hormones like cortisol. This practice can help alleviate physical and mental tension.
2. **Enhanced Mindfulness:** Practicing Tai Chi promotes mindfulness, allowing individuals to cultivate a heightened awareness of the present moment. This mindfulness can reduce rumination and excessive worrying, common contributors to stress.
3. **Improved Physical Health:** Tai Chi improves flexibility, balance, and joint mobility, reducing physical tension and discomfort often

associated with stress.

4. **Emotional Regulation:** Regular practice of Tai Chi can enhance emotional regulation. It provides a safe space to explore and process emotions, leading to greater emotional resilience.

5. **Better Sleep:** Tai Chi has been shown to improve sleep quality. The relaxation and mindfulness developed through Tai Chi can help individuals achieve more restful sleep, even in the face of stress.

6. **Increased Energy:** Tai Chi enhances the flow of energy (Qi) in the body, leaving practitioners feeling invigorated and revitalized, even during challenging times.

7. **Enhanced Coping Skills:** Tai Chi equips individuals with effective coping strategies to manage stress. It fosters a sense of inner calm and adaptability in the face of adversity.

8. **Social Connection:** Group Tai Chi classes provide an opportunity for social interaction and support, which can help reduce feelings of isolation and stress.

9. **Holistic Well-Being:** Tai Chi is a holistic practice that integrates physical, mental, and emotional well-being. It offers a comprehensive approach to stress relief that can positively impact all aspects of your life.

Incorporating Tai Chi into your routine can be a valuable tool for managing stress and promoting overall well-being. It offers a gentle yet powerful way to connect with your body, calm your mind, and develop the resilience needed to navigate life's challenges with grace and equanimity. In the following sections, we will explore Tai Chi techniques and provide guidance on how to integrate this practice into your daily life.

Step-by-Step Instructions for Basic Tai Chi Movements

Tai Chi is renowned for its graceful and flowing movements that promote mindfulness and relaxation. Here are step-by-step instructions for basic Tai Chi movements to help you get started:

1. Wu Ji Stance (Beginning Posture):

- Stand with your feet shoulder-width apart.
- Keep your arms relaxed by your sides, palms facing your thighs.
- Slightly tuck your chin, lengthening your neck.
- Imagine a string pulling you upward from the crown of your head, aligning your spine.
- Close your eyes or maintain a soft gaze, and take a few deep, slow breaths to center yourself.

2. Opening and Closing:

- Inhale as you raise your arms slowly in front of you, palms facing upward.
- Exhale as you lower your arms back down to your sides.
- Repeat this movement, synchronizing your breath with the motion. Imagine gathering and releasing energy with each cycle.

3. Ward Off (Peng):

- Begin in the Wu Ji stance.
- Shift your weight to your right leg as you turn your body slightly to the right.
- Lift your left arm, palm facing forward, and extend your right arm downward.
- As you shift your weight to your left leg, raise your right arm and lower your left arm.
- This creates a circular, spiraling motion.
- Continue this movement in a relaxed and fluid manner, focusing on the flow.

4. Brush Knee (Luo Xi):

- Start in the Wu Ji stance.
- Shift your weight to your right leg and step your left foot forward and to the left at a 45-degree angle.
- As you shift your weight to your left leg, bring your right arm across

your body and your left arm down.

- Rotate your waist and hips to the left.
- Repeat this movement, stepping and brushing in a rhythmic manner.

5. Grasp the Sparrow's Tail (Lan Que Wei):

- Begin in the Wu Ji stance.
- Shift your weight to your right leg.
- Step your left foot to the side and turn your torso slightly to the left.
- As you shift your weight back to your left leg, bring your hands together in front of you, fingers pointing upward.
- Rotate your torso to the right and extend your arms outward, keeping your palms facing forward.
- Imagine gently holding a sparrow in your hands.
- Reverse the movement, shifting your weight and repeating the sequence.

6. Closing Movement:

- To conclude your Tai Chi practice, return to the Wu Ji stance.
- Take a moment to center yourself, close your eyes, and focus on your breath.
- Inhale deeply, and as you exhale, lower your arms to your sides.
- Stand quietly for a few breaths, absorbing the benefits of your practice.

These are basic Tai Chi movements that provide an introduction to the practice. Tai Chi is best learned through observation and guided instruction from a qualified instructor. It's important to maintain a relaxed and flowing motion, synchronize your movements with your breath, and cultivate mindfulness throughout your practice. As you become more familiar with these movements, you can explore longer sequences and forms to deepen your Tai Chi practice and enhance its stress-relieving benefits.

Mindfulness is a powerful practice that can enhance your overall well-being and stress management when incorporated into your daily life. It involves paying deliberate attention to the present moment without judgment. By cultivating mindfulness in everyday activities, you can experience greater presence, reduced stress, and increased resilience. Here's how to integrate mindfulness into various aspects of your daily routine:

1. Mindful Breathing:

- **Morning Routine:** Start your day with a few minutes of mindful breathing. Before getting out of bed, lie on your back, close your eyes, and focus on your breath. Inhale deeply through your nose, exhale through your mouth, and feel the sensations of each breath.
- **During Commutes:** Whether you're driving, biking, or taking public transportation, use your commute as an opportunity to practice mindful breathing. Pay attention to the rhythm of your breath and the sensations of movement.

2. Mindful Eating:

- **Mealtime Ritual:** Set aside time for a dedicated mealtime without distractions. Avoid eating in front of the TV or computer. As you eat, savor each bite, paying attention to the flavors, textures, and aromas of your food.
- **Chew Mindfully:** Chew each bite slowly and thoroughly. Notice the act of chewing and the changes in taste and texture as you break down your food.

3. Mindful Walking:

- **Nature Walk:** Take mindful walks in natural settings like parks or gardens. Pay attention to the sights, sounds, and sensations around you. Feel the ground beneath your feet with each step.
- **Daily Strolls:** During your daily walks, whether for exercise or leisure, practice mindful walking. Be present in your surroundings and let go of any racing thoughts.

4. Mindful Work:

- **Start with Awareness:** As you begin your workday, take a moment to center yourself. Close your eyes and focus on your breath for a few minutes. This can help set a tone of mindfulness for the day.
- **Single-Tasking:** Avoid multitasking and aim to complete one task at a time. Fully engage with the task at hand, whether it's answering emails, writing reports, or attending meetings.

5. Mindful Technology Use:

- **Digital Detox:** Designate specific times for digital detox during the day. Put away your devices and focus on real-world interactions or activities.
- **Mindful Scrolling:** When using social media or browsing the internet, be aware of your intentions and the content you're consuming. Notice how it makes you feel and whether it aligns with your values.

6. Mindful Relationships:

- **Listening Actively:** During conversations, practice active listening. Give the other person your full attention, without thinking about your response or checking your phone.
- **Compassion:** Cultivate empathy and compassion in your interactions. Approach conversations with an open heart and non-judgmental attitude.

7. Mindful Evening Routine:

- **Reflect on the Day:** Before bed, take a few moments to reflect on your day. Acknowledge your accomplishments and challenges without judgment. Consider what you're grateful for.
- **Body Scan:** Lie in bed and perform a body scan by mentally scanning your body from head to toe. Notice any areas of tension or

discomfort and consciously relax them.

8. Mindful Breath Breaks:

- **Throughout the Day:** Set reminders on your phone or computer for short mindful breathing breaks. Take a few deep breaths and bring your awareness to your breath and bodily sensations.

By integrating mindfulness into these everyday activities, you can transform routine moments into opportunities for self-awareness, stress reduction, and personal growth. Mindfulness is a skill that can be developed over time, and with consistent practice, it becomes an integral part of your daily life, helping you navigate stress with greater ease and resilience.

Testimonials from Individuals Who Have Found Peace Through Tai Chi

Tai Chi has touched the lives of countless individuals, bringing them a sense of peace, balance, and well-being. Here are some heartfelt testimonials from people who have experienced the transformative power of Tai Chi in their own words:

Testimonial 1: Sarah's Journey to Inner Peace

Sarah, 54, found herself overwhelmed by the demands of her job and family responsibilities. She shares her Tai Chi journey:

"After a particularly stressful period in my life, I knew I needed a change. That's when I discovered Tai Chi. The gentle, flowing movements and the mindfulness it encouraged were exactly what I needed. Over time, I noticed a profound shift in my inner state. I became more patient, better at handling stress, and more connected to my own body. Tai Chi became my sanctuary, a place where I could find inner peace amidst life's chaos."

Testimonial 2: Michael's Healing Journey

Michael, 63, faced health challenges and emotional trauma. He found solace in Tai Chi:

"I was dealing with health issues and the emotional scars of a difficult past. My journey with Tai Chi started as a way to improve my physical health, but it turned out to be so much more. The practice helped me release pent-up emotions and find a sense of healing. It's like a moving meditation that allowed me to let go of the past and focus on the present. Tai Chi has been an incredible gift on my path to peace and recovery."

Testimonial 3: Emily's Resilience Boost

Emily, 40, was juggling a demanding career and family life. Tai Chi became her anchor:

"Life was throwing curveballs at me left and right. Stress was becoming my constant companion. That's when I decided to try Tai Chi. The practice helped me build resilience like I never imagined. I learned to breathe through challenges, both on and off the mat. It's not about perfection; it's about progress. Tai Chi has given me the tools to navigate life's storms with grace and a deep sense of inner peace."

Testimonial 4: Robert's Quest for Balance

Robert, 68, sought balance and serenity in his retirement years. Tai Chi became his daily ritual:

"Retirement brought its own set of challenges. I wanted to stay active and maintain my mental clarity. Tai Chi came into my life like a breath of fresh air. The slow, deliberate movements grounded me in the present moment. I started each day with Tai Chi, and it set a peaceful tone for everything that followed. It's a practice that keeps me physically and mentally fit while providing a profound sense of inner calm."

Testimonial 5: Grace's Mind-Body Connection

Grace, 58, struggled with anxiety and physical tension. Tai Chi helped her find harmony:

"Anxiety had been a constant companion for years. I could feel the physical tension in my body, and it was taking a toll on my health. Tai Chi introduced me to the mind-body connection like nothing else. The gentle movements and focus on breath

allowed me to release the tension I'd been holding onto. I found a sense of peace and tranquility that had eluded me for so long. Tai Chi has been a true blessing on my journey to holistic well-being."

These heartfelt testimonials reflect the profound impact that Tai Chi can have on one's life. It serves as a reminder that through mindfulness, movement, and a commitment to self-care, individuals can find peace, resilience, and balance even in the midst of life's challenges.

Chapter 8: Holistic Breathwork and Pranayama

Exploring the Significance of Breathwork in Stress Reduction

Breathwork, encompassing practices like Pranayama from the ancient Indian tradition of yoga, holds profound significance in the realm of stress reduction and holistic well-being. In this chapter, we'll dive into why breathwork matters and how it can be a powerful tool for managing stress.

1. The Breath-Body Connection:

Breathing is an inherent aspect of our existence, yet it often goes unnoticed. Breath is the bridge that connects our conscious and unconscious states. By becoming aware of our breath, we can influence both our physiological and psychological well-being.

2. Stress and the Autonomic Nervous System:

Stress triggers the body's "fight or flight" response, activating the sympathetic nervous system. This response can lead to increased heart rate, shallow breathing, and muscle tension. Breathwork offers a way to engage the parasympathetic nervous system, often termed the "rest and digest" system, which promotes relaxation and counteracts the stress response.

3. Mind-Body Harmony:

Breathwork fosters harmony between the mind and body. It encourages mindfulness by anchoring your attention to the present moment—your breath. This simple act of observing and controlling your breath can calm the mind and reduce mental chatter, making it an effective practice for stress management.

4. Stress Reduction Mechanisms:

- **Oxygenation:** Deep, diaphragmatic breathing ensures the body receives an ample supply of oxygen. Well-oxygenated cells function optimally and help alleviate fatigue often associated with stress.

- **Relaxation Response:** Slow, intentional breathwork activates the relaxation response. It lowers blood pressure, reduces muscle tension, and eases anxiety.
- **Mood Regulation:** Breathwork influences the release of neurotransmitters, such as serotonin and dopamine, which play key roles in mood regulation. Consistent breathwork can contribute to a more balanced emotional state.
- **Improved Focus:** Mindful breathing enhances concentration and cognitive function. It allows you to disengage from distractions and stay present in the task at hand, reducing stress related to work or study.
- **Emotional Release:** Breathwork can facilitate the release of suppressed emotions, providing a healthy outlet for emotional processing and reducing the emotional burden of stress.

5. Pranayama in Yoga:

Pranayama is a foundational practice in yoga that focuses on breath control. It acknowledges the life force energy, known as "Prana" in Sanskrit, which is carried and harnessed through the breath. Various Pranayama techniques are designed to influence this energy flow, balancing the mind, body, and spirit.

6. Practical Breathwork Techniques:

- **Deep Abdominal Breathing:** This involves breathing deeply into the diaphragm, expanding the belly with each inhalation and contracting it with each exhalation. It encourages relaxation and reduces shallow chest breathing.
- **Box Breathing:** Inhale for a count of four, hold the breath for four counts, exhale for four counts, and then hold for another four counts before starting the cycle again. This technique calms the nervous system and increases focus.
- **Alternate Nostril Breathing (Nadi Shodhana):** This Pranayama technique involves closing one nostril while inhaling through the other, then switching and exhaling through the opposite nostril. It

balances the right and left hemispheres of the brain, promoting mental clarity and reducing stress.

- **4-7-8 Breathing:** Inhale quietly through your nose for a count of four, hold your breath for a count of seven, and exhale audibly through your mouth for a count of eight. It's a simple but potent technique for relaxation.

Incorporating breathwork and Pranayama into your daily routine can be a transformative practice for stress reduction and holistic well-being. In the following sections of this chapter, we'll delve into specific breathwork techniques, their benefits, and how to integrate them into your life effectively. By harnessing the power of your breath, you can tap into a natural and accessible source of calm and resilience.

Exploring Pranayama Techniques from Different Traditions

Pranayama, the practice of breath control in yoga and other ancient traditions, encompasses a rich tapestry of techniques aimed at harnessing the power of the breath for physical, mental, and spiritual well-being. In this section, we'll introduce various Pranayama techniques from different traditions, each offering its unique benefits:

1. Anulom Vilom (Alternate Nostril Breathing - Yoga):

- Sit comfortably with your spine erect.
- Close your right nostril with your right thumb and inhale deeply through your left nostril.
- Close your left nostril with your right ring finger, release your right nostril, and exhale.
- Inhale through the right nostril.
- Close the right nostril again and exhale through the left nostril.
- Repeat this cycle, alternating nostrils for several minutes.
- Benefits: Balances the left and right hemispheres of the brain, reduces anxiety, and promotes mental clarity.

2. Kapalabhati (Skull Shining Breath - Yoga):

- Sit comfortably with a straight spine and take a deep breath in.
- Exhale forcefully and quickly through your nostrils by contracting your abdominal muscles.
- The inhalation should be passive, and the exhalation should be active.
- Start with a few rounds and gradually increase the speed.
- Benefits: Cleanses the respiratory system, energizes the body, and improves focus.

3. Ujjayi Pranayama (Ocean Breath - Yoga):

- Inhale deeply through your nose.
- Exhale slowly through a slightly constricted throat, producing a soft, audible sound similar to ocean waves.
- Maintain this slight constriction of the throat throughout both inhalation and exhalation.
- Benefits: Relaxes the mind, warms the body, and enhances concentration during yoga practice.

4. Bhramari Pranayama (Humming Bee Breath - Yoga):

- Sit comfortably and close your eyes.
- Place your fingers gently on your closed eyes, index fingers above your eyebrows and other fingers resting on your lower eyelids.
- Take a deep breath in and, as you exhale, make a humming sound like a bee.
- Continue for several breaths, feeling the vibrations in your head.
- Benefits: Calms the mind, relieves stress, and soothes the nervous system.

5. Box Breathing (Militaristic Tradition):

- Sit or stand comfortably with a straight spine.
- Inhale deeply through your nose for a count of four.
- Hold your breath for a count of four.
- Exhale through your nose for a count of four.

- Hold your breath again for a count of four.
- Repeat this cycle for several rounds.
- Benefits: Reduces anxiety, enhances focus, and stabilizes the nervous system.

6. Qigong Breathing (Chinese Tradition):

- Stand or sit comfortably with a straight spine.
- Inhale gently through your nose, filling your lower abdomen first and then your chest.
- Exhale slowly and completely, releasing tension.
- Maintain a calm and even rhythm.
- Benefits: Promotes Qi (vital energy) flow, improves lung capacity, and cultivates a sense of inner peace.

7. Sama Vritti (Equal Breathing - Yogic and Mindfulness Traditions):

- Sit in a comfortable position with an upright spine.
- Inhale and exhale for an equal count, such as inhaling for a count of four and exhaling for a count of four.
- Gradually increase the count as you become more comfortable.
- Benefits: Enhances concentration, balances the nervous system, and reduces stress.

These Pranayama techniques, drawn from diverse traditions, offer versatile tools for harnessing the transformative potential of your breath. Whether you seek relaxation, mental clarity, or heightened awareness, incorporating these practices into your daily routine can lead to profound benefits for your holistic well-being and stress reduction. In the following sections of this chapter, we will explore these techniques in more detail and provide guidance on their practical application in your life.

Practical Exercises to Enhance Breath Awareness

Enhancing your breath awareness is a fundamental step in harnessing the benefits of breathwork and Pranayama. By developing a deeper connection with your breath, you can unlock its potential to reduce stress and promote overall well-being. Here are some practical exercises to help you cultivate breath awareness:

1. Full Abdominal Breathing:

- Sit or lie down in a comfortable position.
- Place one hand on your chest and the other on your abdomen.
- Take a slow, deep breath in through your nose, allowing your abdomen to rise as you fill your lungs.
- Exhale slowly through your mouth, feeling your abdomen fall.
- Continue this practice for several breaths, focusing on the rise and fall of your abdomen with each breath.
- **Benefits:** This exercise promotes deep diaphragmatic breathing, which is calming and helps reduce stress.

2. Breath Counting:

- Find a quiet space to sit comfortably.
- Close your eyes and take a few natural breaths to settle in.
- Begin counting your breaths, starting with "one" as you inhale, "two" as you exhale, and so on.
- Continue counting up to a specific number, such as ten, and then start again from one.
- If your mind wanders or you lose count, gently return your focus to your breath and start over.
- **Benefits:** This exercise enhances concentration and awareness of the breath.

3. Triangle Breathing:

- Visualize an equilateral triangle in your mind, with one point at the top and two at the bottom.
- Inhale slowly as you trace one side of the triangle upward in your mind's eye.

- Hold your breath briefly as you reach the top point of the triangle.
- Exhale slowly as you trace the other two sides of the triangle downward.
- Pause briefly at the bottom before beginning the next cycle.
- Repeat this visualization for several breath cycles.
- **Benefits:** Triangle breathing encourages a deliberate and balanced breath pattern, fostering relaxation and mental clarity.

4. Sensory Breath Awareness:

- Sit quietly and close your eyes.
- Direct your attention to the sensation of your breath as it enters and exits your nostrils.
- Notice the temperature, texture, and flow of the breath at the entrance of your nostrils.
- Pay attention to any subtle sensations in this area.
- Continue to focus on the sensation of your breath for a few minutes.
- **Benefits:** This exercise enhances sensory awareness and promotes mindfulness of the breath.

5. Breath Observation in Nature:

- Find a peaceful outdoor setting, such as a park or garden.
- Sit or stand comfortably and observe your natural surroundings.
- Notice how the wind moves through trees, causing leaves to rustle.
- Observe the ebb and flow of your breath in harmony with the natural world.
- Feel the connection between your breath and the environment.
- **Benefits:** This exercise promotes a sense of oneness with nature and deepens breath awareness.

Regular practice of these exercises can help you develop a heightened sense of breath awareness. This heightened awareness becomes a valuable tool for stress reduction and can be seamlessly integrated into your daily life. In the upcoming sections, we will delve deeper into specific Pranayama techniques and their applications to further enhance your holistic well-being.

Integrating Breathwork into Daily Routines

Breathwork is most effective when it becomes an integral part of your daily life. By seamlessly weaving breath awareness and Pranayama techniques into your routines, you can harness their stress-reducing and holistic benefits. Here's how you can integrate breathwork into your daily activities:

1. Morning Awakening:

- **Start your day with intention:** Before getting out of bed, take a few minutes for deep, mindful breaths. Inhale positivity and exhale any residual sleepiness or tension.
- **Mindful Shower:** During your morning shower, take a moment to focus on your breath. Feel the warm water on your skin and synchronize your breath with the flow of water, allowing it to wash away any mental or physical heaviness.

2. Commute and Transportation:

- **Traffic Breath:** If you're driving or stuck in traffic, utilize this time to practice deep breathing. Inhale calmness and exhale any frustration or impatience.
- **Public Transport Breathing:** During bus, train, or subway rides, use the rhythmic motion as a cue for breath awareness. Inhale with the sway or motion, exhale with the next movement.

3. Work and Study:

- **Desk Reset:** Set reminders to pause and take a few mindful breaths throughout your work or study day. These mini-breaks can enhance focus and reduce stress.
- **Meeting Preparation:** Before important meetings or presentations,

practice calming breathwork to steady your nerves and boost your confidence.

4. Mealtime Ritual:

- **Mindful Eating:** Prior to eating, pause to take a few mindful breaths. This practice encourages present-moment awareness and helps you savor your food fully.
- **Chew and Breathe:** During meals, chew each bite deliberately and take a breath between bites. This not only aids digestion but also prevents overeating.

5. Exercise and Physical Activity:

- **Pre-Exercise Breathing:** Before your workout or yoga session, engage in Pranayama to prepare your body and mind. Deep breaths can optimize your exercise routine.
- **Breath Synchronization:** During physical activities, synchronize your breath with your movements. This can enhance your performance and reduce the perception of effort.

6. Mindful Breaks:

- **Scheduled Breathing Breaks:** Set specific times during the day for mindful breathing breaks. These can be moments of quiet reflection and relaxation, even if just for a few minutes.
- **Nature Connection:** Whenever possible, take short walks outdoors and align your breath with the natural rhythms of the environment. Feel the interconnectedness of your breath with the world around you.

7. Evening Wind Down:

- **Screen Time Transition:** As you transition away from screens in the evening, engage in calming Pranayama to signal your body that it's time to relax.

- **Bedtime Breath:** Before sleep, practice deep, slow breaths to calm your mind and prepare your body for restful slumber.

8. Social Interactions:

- **Listening Breath:** During conversations with friends or loved ones, maintain a mindful breath to truly listen and respond with presence and empathy.
- **Pause and Reflect:** In social situations, take short, silent breath pauses to center yourself and maintain composure.

Integrating breathwork into your daily routines doesn't require significant time or effort. It's about making a conscious choice to infuse mindfulness and Pranayama into the moments that matter most to you. Over time, this practice becomes second nature, helping you navigate life's challenges with grace, resilience, and a profound sense of inner calm. In the following sections, we will explore specific Pranayama techniques in more detail, offering guidance on their practical application in various aspects of your life.

Personal Stories of Transformation Through Breathwork

Breathwork and Pranayama have the remarkable capacity to catalyze transformative experiences in individuals. These stories from real people illustrate how the power of breath can create profound shifts in one's life:

Story 1: Maria's Journey to Inner Healing

Maria, a 42-year-old survivor of trauma, shares her transformative experience with breathwork:

"I carried the weight of my past trauma for years, and it felt like an unbreakable chain. A friend introduced me to breathwork as a way to heal. At first, it was challenging, but as I persisted, I began to feel sensations and emotions I had buried deep within. The breath became a bridge to my healing. Each conscious inhale and exhale helped me release the pain and find a sense of peace I hadn't known in years.

Breathwork allowed me to rewrite my story and heal from the inside out. It was a profound transformation, and I am forever grateful."

Story 2: John's Journey from Anxiety to Calm

John, a 34-year-old marketing executive, describes how breathwork transformed his life:

"I was constantly on edge due to the pressures of my job and the fast pace of modern life. Stress and anxiety were my constant companions. I decided to explore breathwork as a last resort. Through guided sessions, I learned to regulate my breath and become aware of my thoughts and emotions. Slowly but surely, my anxiety began to lose its grip. I felt a sense of calm I hadn't experienced in years. The breath became my anchor, helping me navigate high-stress situations with poise and confidence. Breathwork was my game-changer, and it continues to be my source of inner strength."

Story 3: Sarah's Journey to Mind-Body Harmony

Sarah, a 28-year-old yoga instructor, shares her journey of integrating breathwork into her practice:

"Yoga was always a physical practice for me until I discovered the power of Pranayama. It was during a challenging time in my life when I realized that my breath could be my greatest ally. As I deepened my Pranayama practice, I unlocked a new level of mind-body connection. The breath became a bridge between my physical and spiritual self. It was in those moments of deep, intentional breathing that I felt the unity of body, mind, and soul. Breathwork transformed my yoga practice from a mere workout to a spiritual journey. It has opened up a world of inner exploration and self-discovery that continues to unfold."

Story 4: James's Journey to Resilience

James, a 50-year-old entrepreneur, recounts how breathwork helped him navigate life's challenges:

"Running my business was a rollercoaster of stress and uncertainty. I often felt overwhelmed and burnt out. Then I stumbled upon breathwork as a tool for

resilience. It wasn't an instant fix, but as I incorporated breathwork into my daily life, I noticed a gradual shift. The breath became my anchor in the storm of entrepreneurship. It helped me stay centered during high-pressure meetings and make clearer decisions. It taught me that I could weather any storm with grace. Breathwork has made me a more resilient leader, husband, and father."

Story 5: Emily's Journey to Self-Discovery

Emily, a 30-year-old artist, shares how breathwork led her on a journey of self-discovery:

"As an artist, I was often in my head, overthinking and doubting my creativity. Breathwork entered my life as a catalyst for self-exploration. Through deep breaths, I learned to silence the inner critic and embrace my artistic intuition. The breath became my muse, guiding me to uncharted creative territories. It was in those moments of surrender to the breath that I discovered my true artistic voice. Breathwork unlocked a wellspring of creativity within me, and it continues to be my well of inspiration."

These personal stories illustrate the transformative potential of breathwork and Pranayama in different aspects of life. Whether for healing, stress reduction, self-discovery, or resilience, the breath serves as a powerful tool for personal growth and holistic well-being. As you embark on your own breathwork journey, remember that your breath has the capacity to bring about profound and positive changes in your life.

Chapter 9: Creating Holistic Lifestyle Habits

Exploring the Importance of Consistency and Sustainability in Holistic Practices

In the journey of embracing holistic practices for stress management, the significance of consistency and sustainability cannot be overstated. These two pillars form the foundation upon which lasting positive change is built. Let's delve into why they are crucial and how they contribute to your holistic well-being:

1. Building Resilience Through Consistency:

- **Mind-Body Connection:** Consistent holistic practices, whether it's yoga, meditation, or breathwork, foster a strong mind-body connection. Just as exercising a muscle makes it stronger, regular engagement with these practices strengthens your mental and physical resilience.
- **Stress Response:** Consistency trains your body and mind to respond more calmly to stressors. Over time, the stress response becomes less reactive, reducing the impact of daily challenges on your overall well-being.
- **Neuroplasticity:** Consistent mindfulness practices, such as meditation, promote neuroplasticity—the brain's ability to rewire itself. This can lead to enduring changes in how you perceive and respond to stress.

2. Sustainable Practices for Long-Term Benefits:

- **Aligning with Your Lifestyle:** Sustainability in holistic practices means finding approaches that seamlessly fit into your daily life. When these practices become a natural part of your routine, they are more likely to endure.
- **Avoiding Burnout:** Sustainable practices are those that you can

maintain without feeling overwhelmed or exhausted. Burnout can occur if you push yourself too hard or adopt practices that are not feasible in the long run.

- **Holistic Nutrition:** Sustainable nutrition choices involve adopting a balanced and nourishing diet that you can sustain over time. Extreme diets or restrictions often lead to short-term results but are challenging to maintain.

3. The Compound Effect of Consistency:

- **Small Steps, Big Changes:** Consistency magnifies the impact of small daily actions. Over time, these seemingly insignificant practices accumulate and create a substantial shift in your overall well-being.
- **Holistic Nutrition:** Consistently choosing wholesome foods nourishes your body on a cellular level. The compound effect of a nutrient-rich diet can improve energy levels, mental clarity, and resilience to stress.

4. Balancing Progress and Patience:

- **Recognizing Progress:** Consistency helps you recognize gradual progress. It's not always about immediate results but the steady journey toward holistic well-being.
- **Embracing Patience:** Sustainable practices require patience. Realizing that change takes time can reduce frustration and discouragement on your path to managing stress holistically.

5. Creating a Holistic Lifestyle Blueprint:

- **Routine Integration:** Sustainable holistic practices become integrated into your daily routine. They seamlessly coexist with your work, family, and social life, making it easier to prioritize self-care.
- **Personalization:** The most sustainable practices are those tailored to your unique needs and preferences. Embrace practices that resonate

with you, ensuring they become a natural part of your lifestyle.

6. The Domino Effect of Consistency:

- **Positive Habits Multiply:** Consistency in one area of holistic wellness often leads to positive changes in others. For example, regular yoga practice might inspire you to explore meditation or conscious breathing.
- **Mindful Awareness:** Consistency fosters mindful awareness of your choices and their impact on your well-being. This awareness naturally extends to other areas of your life.

Consistency and sustainability in holistic practices form the bedrock of a resilient and balanced lifestyle. By committing to regular engagement with these practices and choosing approaches that align with your unique needs and circumstances, you create a holistic lifestyle blueprint that can withstand the test of time. In the chapters that follow, we will explore specific holistic practices and offer guidance on how to incorporate them into your life consistently and sustainably. Remember that it's the journey of self-discovery and well-being that matters, and that journey is best traveled with patience, self-compassion, and a commitment to holistic living.

Guidance on Building a Daily Routine that Includes Holistic Stress Management

Building a daily routine that incorporates holistic stress management practices can be a transformative journey toward greater well-being. Here's a step-by-step guide to help you create a balanced and sustainable daily routine:

1. Set Clear Intentions:

- **Start with a Vision:** Begin by envisioning the kind of day you want to have. What does a stress-resilient and balanced day look like to you?
- **Define Your Priorities:** Identify the holistic practices that matter most to you. These might include yoga, meditation, breathwork, or

mindfulness.

2. Morning Rituals:

- **Mindful Awakening:** Start your day with a moment of mindfulness. As you wake up, take a few deep breaths, expressing gratitude for the new day ahead.
- **Morning Movement:** Incorporate gentle movement into your morning routine, such as stretching or yoga. This helps awaken your body and mind.

3. Mindful Breakfast:

- **Nourishing Nutrition:** Choose a balanced and nourishing breakfast that sets a positive tone for the day. Include whole grains, fruits, and proteins.
- **Mindful Eating:** Practice mindful eating by savoring each bite, paying attention to textures and flavors. This promotes conscious nourishment.

4. Work and Productivity:

- **Breath Breaks:** Integrate short breath breaks throughout your workday. Every hour, pause for a few moments of deep breathing to reset and refocus.
- **Mindful Work:** Approach tasks with mindfulness, one at a time. Complete each task before moving on to the next, reducing stress associated with multitasking.

5. Midday Recharge:

- **Lunchtime Wellness:** Dedicate a portion of your lunch break to holistic practices. You can do a short meditation, take a walk, or practice Pranayama.
- **Hydration:** Stay hydrated by sipping water throughout the day.

Proper hydration supports physical and mental well-being.

6. Afternoon Resilience:

- **Mindful Movement:** In the afternoon, engage in mindful movement. This could be a brief yoga session or a walk outdoors to re-energize your body and mind.
- **Stress Awareness:** Take a moment to assess your stress levels and acknowledge any challenges. Awareness is the first step in managing stress effectively.

7. Evening Rituals:

- **Digital Detox:** Start winding down by disconnecting from screens at least an hour before bedtime. This supports restful sleep.
- **Relaxation Practices:** Engage in relaxation practices like meditation or breathwork in the evening. These practices prepare your mind and body for rest.

8. Restorative Sleep:

- **Sleep Hygiene:** Prioritize quality sleep by creating a conducive sleep environment. Ensure your room is dark, quiet, and at a comfortable temperature.
- **Consistent Sleep Schedule:** Maintain a regular sleep schedule by going to bed and waking up at the same times each day. Consistency supports a well-rested body and mind.

9. Reflection and Gratitude:

- **Daily Reflection:** Before sleep, take a moment to reflect on your day. Acknowledge your achievements and identify areas for improvement.
- **Gratitude Practice:** Express gratitude for the positive aspects of your day. Cultivating gratitude fosters a positive outlook and reduces stress.

10. Adapt and Refine:

- **Flexibility:** Your daily routine should be adaptable to accommodate unforeseen events. Embrace flexibility while staying committed to your holistic practices.
- **Continuous Learning:** Be open to refining your routine over time. As you discover what works best for you, make adjustments to optimize your well-being.

Remember that building a holistic daily routine is a process, and it's okay to start small. Gradually introduce new practices and allow yourself the grace of imperfection. Your routine should be a source of support and empowerment, not an additional source of stress. By consistently and mindfully incorporating holistic stress management practices into your daily life, you can cultivate resilience, inner calm, and holistic well-being.

The Role of Sleep, Hydration, and Physical Activity in Stress Resilience

Achieving stress resilience extends beyond specific holistic practices; it encompasses fundamental aspects of daily life. Sleep, hydration, and physical activity are key pillars that significantly influence your ability to manage stress effectively. Here's an exploration of their roles in enhancing stress resilience:

1. Sleep: The Foundation of Resilience

- **Quality vs. Quantity:** It's not just about the number of hours you sleep but the quality of your sleep that matters. Restorative sleep allows your body and mind to recover, reducing stress levels.
- **Stress Hormone Regulation:** Adequate sleep regulates stress hormones like cortisol. Disrupted sleep patterns can lead to increased stress reactivity.
- **Emotional Balance:** Sleep plays a crucial role in emotional regulation. A well-rested mind is better equipped to handle stress and emotional challenges.
- **Cognitive Function:** Quality sleep enhances cognitive functions

such as decision-making, problem-solving, and memory, which are essential for effective stress management.

Tips for Better Sleep:

- Create a consistent sleep schedule.
- Establish a relaxing bedtime routine.
- Ensure a comfortable sleep environment.
- Limit screen time before bedtime.
- Avoid caffeine and heavy meals close to bedtime.

2. Hydration: Nourishing Body and Mind

- **Brain Function:** Hydration is essential for optimal brain function. Dehydration can impair cognitive performance and increase stress.
- **Stress Reduction:** Staying hydrated supports the body's natural stress response. Dehydration can lead to increased cortisol levels and heightened stress.
- **Physical Well-Being:** Proper hydration aids in maintaining physical health, which is closely linked to stress resilience. Dehydration can lead to physical stress on the body.
- **Mood Stability:** Dehydration can contribute to mood swings and irritability, making it harder to cope with stressors.

Tips for Staying Hydrated:

- Drink water consistently throughout the day.
- Monitor your urine color to gauge hydration levels.
- Include hydrating foods like fruits and vegetables in your diet.
- Avoid excessive caffeine and alcohol, which can lead to dehydration.

3. Physical Activity: Stress Relief through Movement

- **Stress Hormone Regulation:** Physical activity, such as regular exercise or mindful movement practices like yoga or Tai Chi, helps regulate stress hormones and reduces cortisol levels.

- **Endorphin Release:** Exercise stimulates the release of endorphins, the body's natural mood lifters. These can counteract the effects of stress.
- **Mind-Body Connection:** Movement practices like yoga and Tai Chi enhance the mind-body connection, promoting relaxation and reducing stress.
- **Improved Sleep:** Regular physical activity can lead to better sleep quality, contributing to overall stress resilience.

Tips for Incorporating Physical Activity:

- Find an activity you enjoy, whether it's walking, dancing, or sports.
- Aim for at least 150 minutes of moderate-intensity exercise per week.
- Include both aerobic and strength-training exercises in your routine.
- Practice mindful movement for stress reduction and flexibility.

Incorporating these fundamental elements—quality sleep, proper hydration, and regular physical activity—into your daily life creates a strong foundation for stress resilience. They support your body and mind in effectively managing stressors and enhancing overall well-being. As you cultivate these holistic lifestyle habits, you'll find yourself better equipped to face life's challenges with grace and resilience.

Strategies for Overcoming Obstacles and Setbacks

On the journey to holistic stress management and well-being, obstacles and setbacks are natural and expected. What truly matters is how you navigate these challenges and continue moving forward. Here are strategies to help you overcome obstacles and setbacks effectively:

1. Cultivate Resilience:

- **Mindset Shift:** Embrace setbacks as opportunities for growth rather than failures. See them as valuable lessons on your path to holistic well-being.

- **Learn and Adapt:** Reflect on the reasons behind the setback. What can you learn from it? Use this knowledge to adjust your approach and make more informed choices.

2. Set Realistic Expectations:

- **Avoid Perfectionism:** Understand that holistic practices, like any other aspect of life, have ups and downs. Strive for progress, not perfection.
- **Small Steps:** Break down your goals into smaller, achievable steps. Celebrate each milestone to stay motivated.

3. Maintain Self-Compassion:

- **Positive Self-Talk:** Be mindful of your self-talk. Replace self-criticism with self-compassion. Treat yourself as kindly as you would a dear friend facing similar challenges.
- **Acknowledge Emotions:** It's okay to feel frustrated, disappointed, or discouraged at times. Allow yourself to experience these emotions without judgment.

4. Seek Support and Guidance:

- **Community:** Connect with like-minded individuals who share your holistic well-being goals. Join support groups, forums, or classes to build a sense of community.
- **Mentorship:** Consider seeking guidance from a mentor or coach who specializes in holistic practices. Their experience can provide valuable insights and encouragement.

5. Mindful Self-Reflection:

- **Journaling:** Keep a journal to document your journey, including both successes and setbacks. Journaling can help you identify patterns and make adjustments.

- **Regular Check-Ins:** Take time for introspection. Regularly assess your progress, challenges, and areas for improvement.

6. Flexibility and Adaptation:

- **Embrace Change:** Be open to adapting your holistic practices as needed. What worked for you in the past may not be the best fit for your current circumstances.
- **Explore Alternatives:** If one practice or approach doesn't yield the desired results, explore alternative methods or holistic practices that align better with your needs.

7. Patience and Persistence:

- **Long-Term Perspective:** Keep in mind that holistic well-being is a lifelong journey. Temporary setbacks do not define your overall progress.
- **Celebrate Progress:** Celebrate your achievements, no matter how small. Recognize the effort you put into your well-being.

8. Mindfulness and Stress Reduction:

- **Stress Management Tools:** Utilize the holistic stress management tools you've learned, such as meditation, breathwork, or mindfulness, to navigate setbacks with composure.
- **Coping Strategies:** Apply stress reduction techniques to manage the emotional and physical effects of setbacks effectively.

9. Reframe Setbacks as Opportunities:

- **Growth Mindset:** Embrace a growth mindset that views challenges as opportunities for personal development and transformation.
- **Reevaluate Priorities:** Setbacks can prompt you to reassess your priorities and make more aligned choices in your holistic journey.

10. Stay Committed:

- **Renew Your Commitment:** Remind yourself of the reasons why you embarked on the path of holistic well-being. Reconnect with your sense of purpose and commitment.
- **Consistency Matters:** Even during setbacks, maintain some level of consistency in your holistic practices. This continuity can help you regain momentum.

Remember that setbacks are part of the journey to holistic well-being. They do not diminish your progress but rather offer opportunities for resilience, growth, and self-discovery. By applying these strategies and approaching setbacks with a compassionate and determined mindset, you can continue on your path to holistic stress management with greater strength and clarity.

Holistic Lifestyle Tips for Long-Term Well-Being

Long-term well-being is the ultimate goal of adopting holistic practices for stress management. Here are some holistic lifestyle tips to support your journey towards lasting health and well-being:

1. Prioritize Self-Care:

- **Daily Self-Care:** Make self-care an essential part of your daily routine. Prioritize it just as you would any other commitment.
- **Unplug Regularly:** Set aside time to disconnect from digital devices and screens. This allows for mental and emotional rejuvenation.

2. Nourish Your Body:

- **Balanced Diet:** Maintain a well-balanced diet rich in whole foods, including fruits, vegetables, lean proteins, and whole grains.
- **Mindful Eating:** Practice mindful eating by savoring each bite and paying attention to your body's hunger and fullness cues.

3. Stay Active and Mindful:

- **Regular Exercise:** Incorporate regular physical activity into your life. Find activities you enjoy, whether it's yoga, walking, dancing, or playing a sport.
- **Mindful Movement:** Engage in mindful movement practices like yoga, Tai Chi, or Qigong. These enhance your mind-body connection and reduce stress.

4. Rest and Recovery:

- **Prioritize Sleep:** Ensure you get adequate and restorative sleep. Maintain a consistent sleep schedule to support your body's natural rhythms.
- **Rest Days:** Schedule regular rest days to allow your body and mind to recover from physical and mental exertion.

5. Practice Gratitude:

- **Gratitude Journal:** Keep a gratitude journal to regularly reflect on the positive aspects of your life. Cultivating gratitude fosters a positive outlook.
- **Express Thanks:** Take the time to express gratitude to the people who enhance your life. It strengthens your relationships and promotes well-being.

6. Mindfulness and Stress Reduction:

- **Daily Practice:** Dedicate time to daily mindfulness practices like meditation, breathwork, or progressive muscle relaxation.
- **Stress Awareness:** Continuously assess your stress levels and make adjustments to your routine to reduce stressors.

7. Seek Connection:

- **Social Support:** Foster meaningful connections with friends and family. Social support is essential for emotional well-being.

- **Community Engagement:** Get involved in community activities or volunteer work. Contribution to a larger community can bring a sense of purpose.

8. Lifelong Learning:

- **Continued Growth:** Cultivate a lifelong learning mindset. Embrace new experiences, skills, and knowledge to promote mental and emotional well-being.
- **Set Goals:** Set and pursue personal and professional goals that align with your values and passions.

9. Nature Connection:

- **Time in Nature:** Spend time in natural settings whenever possible. Nature has a calming and restorative effect on the mind and body.
- **Mindful Nature:** Practice mindfulness in nature by observing the sights, sounds, and sensations around you.

10. Stress-Reduction Techniques:

- **Stress Management Toolbox:** Build a toolbox of stress-reduction techniques, including yoga, aromatherapy, herbal remedies, and holistic nutrition.
- **Regular Check-Ins:** Routinely assess your stress management practices and make adjustments as needed to enhance their effectiveness.

11. Holistic Healthcare:

- **Consult Professionals:** When seeking guidance for holistic practices like herbal remedies, consult with qualified herbalists or healthcare professionals.
- **Open Communication:** Maintain open communication with your healthcare provider about your holistic practices to ensure safe and

effective integration.

12. Balance and Adaptability:

- **Balance Your Life:** Strive for balance in all aspects of your life, including work, relationships, and self-care.
- **Adapt to Change:** Embrace change as a natural part of life. Be flexible and adaptable in the face of challenges.

Remember that holistic well-being is a lifelong journey, and it's the consistency and commitment to these holistic lifestyle tips that will contribute to your long-term health and happiness. Each day is an opportunity to nurture your body, mind, and spirit, and by doing so, you create a foundation for a vibrant and fulfilling life.

Chapter 10: Integrating Holistic Practices into Your Life

Summarizing Key Takeaways from Previous Chapters

As you embark on your journey of integrating holistic practices into your life for stress management and well-being, it's essential to revisit and reflect on the key takeaways from the previous chapters. These insights serve as a roadmap for your holistic well-being journey:

Chapter 1: Understanding Stress

- Stress is a natural response to life's challenges, but chronic stress can harm physical and mental health.
- Recognizing stressors and their impact is the first step in managing stress effectively.
- Proactively managing stress is vital for holistic well-being.

Chapter 2: Yoga for Stress Relief

- Yoga offers profound physical and mental benefits for stress reduction.
- Basic yoga poses and breathing exercises can be integrated into your routine.
- Real-life success stories highlight the transformative power of yoga.

Chapter 3: The Power of Meditation

- Meditation positively impacts the brain and emotional well-being.
- Various meditation techniques, including mindfulness and loving-kindness, provide versatile tools for stress reduction.
- Creating a peaceful meditation space and addressing common challenges are crucial for meditation practice.

Chapter 4: Aromatherapy for Stress Reduction

- Aromatherapy uses essential oils to influence mood and relaxation.
- DIY aromatherapy blends offer a personalized approach to stress management.
- Safety precautions and case studies demonstrate the benefits of aromatherapy.

Chapter 5: Herbal Remedies and Adaptogens

- Adaptogens play a key role in stress management.
- Specific herbs and adaptogenic plants like ashwagandha and ginseng have stress-reducing properties.
- Recipes for herbal teas and tinctures provide holistic solutions.

Chapter 6: Holistic Nutrition for Stress Resilience

- Diet significantly affects stress levels.
- Certain foods exacerbate stress, while others alleviate it.
- Holistic nutrition includes meal planning, hydration, and balanced nutrition.

Chapter 7: Mindful Movement and Tai Chi

- Tai Chi is a mindful movement practice with numerous stress-relief benefits.
- Principles of Tai Chi enhance well-being.
- Testimonials emphasize the transformative power of Tai Chi.

Chapter 8: Holistic Breathwork and Pranayama

- Breathwork is a powerful tool for stress reduction.
- Pranayama techniques from various traditions offer versatile options.
- Breath awareness exercises and personal stories illustrate its impact.

Chapter 9: Creating Holistic Lifestyle Habits

- Consistency and sustainability are key to holistic practices.

- Building a daily routine that includes holistic stress management is essential.
- Sleep, hydration, and physical activity play vital roles in stress resilience.

Chapter 10: Integrating Holistic Practices into Your Life

- Reflect on and apply the key takeaways from each chapter.
- Embrace setbacks as opportunities for growth.
- Prioritize self-care, nourish your body, and practice gratitude.
- Maintain a holistic approach to well-being, balancing physical, mental, and emotional health.

By integrating these insights into your daily life, you embark on a holistic well-being journey that fosters resilience, inner peace, and long-term health. Remember that your holistic path is unique, and it's the consistent, mindful application of these principles that will lead to lasting transformation and well-being.

Creating Your Personalized Holistic Stress Management Toolkit

As you conclude this journey towards holistic stress management and well-being, it's time to assemble a personalized toolkit. This toolkit will serve as your go-to resource for managing stress holistically. Here's how you can create your own:

1. Mindfulness and Meditation Practices:

- **Mindful Breathing:** Incorporate daily breath awareness exercises to stay present and calm.
- **Meditation:** Choose a meditation technique that resonates with you, whether it's mindfulness, loving-kindness, or guided meditation.
- **Meditation Space:** Create a serene meditation space at home where you can retreat for moments of inner peace.

2. Yoga and Mindful Movement:

- **Yoga Poses:** Select a few yoga poses that you enjoy and that target stress relief.
- **Tai Chi or Qigong:** Integrate mindful movement practices like Tai Chi or Qigong into your routine.
- **Daily Stretching:** Incorporate a few minutes of stretching throughout the day to release tension.

3. Aromatherapy and Essential Oils:

- **Essential Oils:** Identify essential oils that resonate with you for relaxation and stress relief.
- **Aromatherapy Blends:** Create DIY aromatherapy blends or purchase pre-made blends for various situations.
- **Diffuser:** Invest in a diffuser to disperse calming scents throughout your living space.

4. Herbal Remedies and Adaptogens:

- **Adaptogenic Herbs:** Explore adaptogens like ashwagandha or ginseng to support stress resilience.
- **Herbal Teas:** Craft a collection of stress-relieving herbal teas for different times of the day.
- **Consultation:** If using herbs medicinally, consult an herbalist or healthcare professional for guidance.

5. Holistic Nutrition:

- **Balanced Diet:** Design a balanced meal plan rich in stress-reducing foods.
- **Hydration:** Create a daily hydration goal and track your water intake.
- **Meal Prep:** Dedicate time for meal preparation to ensure nourishing, stress-reducing meals.

6. Holistic Breathwork and Pranayama:

- **Breathing Exercises:** Select pranayama techniques that resonate with you, such as diaphragmatic breathing or alternate nostril breathing.
- **Breath Awareness:** Practice daily breath awareness exercises to stay centered and calm.
- **Integration:** Incorporate breathwork into your routine during moments of stress or as part of your meditation practice.

7. Holistic Lifestyle Habits:

- **Self-Care Rituals:** Establish daily self-care rituals that nurture your body, mind, and spirit.
- **Sleep Routine:** Create a consistent sleep schedule and prioritize sleep hygiene for restorative rest.
- **Daily Routine:** Craft a daily routine that includes holistic practices, self-reflection, and gratitude.

8. Stress-Reduction Strategies:

- **Stress Journal:** Keep a stress journal to identify triggers and patterns.
- **Support Network:** Cultivate a support network of friends, family, or like-minded individuals.
- **Professional Guidance:** Seek guidance from holistic practitioners, therapists, or coaches as needed.

9. Mindful Technology Use:

- **Digital Detox:** Schedule regular breaks from screens and digital devices.
- **Mindful Consumption:** Consume digital content mindfully, focusing on what enhances your well-being.

10. Adapt and Personalize:

- **Flexibility:** Remain open to adjusting your toolkit as your needs change.

- **Personalization:** Tailor your toolkit to your unique preferences and circumstances.

Remember that your holistic stress management toolkit is a dynamic resource. It evolves with you as you learn and grow on your journey towards well-being. Regularly revisit and refine it to ensure that it continues to serve you effectively in managing stress and promoting holistic health. Your personalized toolkit is a powerful ally on your path to lasting well-being and resilience.

Setting Achievable Goals and Tracking Progress

Creating achievable goals and tracking your progress is essential for successful integration of holistic practices into your life for stress management. Here are some tips to help you set meaningful goals and monitor your journey effectively:

1. Start with Clarity:

- **Define Your Why:** Clearly articulate why you want to incorporate holistic practices into your life. Understanding your motivations helps maintain commitment.
- **Identify Specific Goals:** Break down your broader goal into specific, actionable objectives. For example, if your goal is to reduce stress, specify how you plan to achieve this through yoga, meditation, or other practices.

2. SMART Goals:

- **Specific:** Ensure your goals are clear and well-defined. Instead of saying, "I want to meditate more," specify, "I will meditate for 15 minutes every morning."
- **Measurable:** Set goals that can be quantified. It's easier to track progress when you have specific metrics. For instance, "I will drink eight glasses of water daily."
- **Achievable:** Ensure your goals are realistic and attainable. Consider

your current commitments and available resources when setting goals.

- **Relevant:** Align your goals with your values and priorities. Make sure they genuinely contribute to your well-being.
- **Time-Bound:** Set a timeframe for your goals. Having a deadline creates a sense of urgency and accountability. For example, "I will practice yoga three times a week for three months."

3. Break It Down:

- **Chunk Goals:** If your holistic journey involves multiple practices, break them down into smaller, manageable steps. This prevents overwhelm.
- **Weekly Goals:** Set weekly goals that lead to your larger, long-term objectives. These smaller milestones keep you on track.

4. Document Your Goals:

- **Write It Down:** Document your goals in a journal or digital note. This makes them tangible and reinforces your commitment.
- **Visual Aids:** Create a vision board or use visual aids to represent your goals. Visualization can enhance motivation.

5. Daily or Weekly Tracking:

- **Journaling:** Maintain a progress journal to record your daily or weekly achievements, insights, and challenges. Reflect on how each practice impacts your well-being.
- **Checklists:** Use checklists to track your daily or weekly holistic practices. Checking off completed tasks provides a sense of accomplishment.

6. Set Reminders:

- **Digital Reminders:** Utilize digital tools like alarms, calendar alerts, or habit-tracking apps to remind you of your daily practices.

- **Physical Reminders:** Place visual cues, such as post-it notes or meaningful objects, in your environment to prompt mindfulness of your goals.

7. Celebrate Achievements:

- **Reward Yourself:** Celebrate your achievements, whether big or small. Treat yourself to something special or engage in a self-care ritual.
- **Acknowledge Progress:** Regularly review your progress and acknowledge how far you've come. This boosts motivation and self-esteem.

8. Seek Accountability:

- **Accountability Partner:** Share your goals with a trusted friend or family member who can help keep you on track and provide encouragement.
- **Join a Group:** Consider joining a holistic well-being group or class where you can share your goals and progress with like-minded individuals.

9. Adapt and Learn:

- **Flexibility:** Be open to adjusting your goals as needed. Life circumstances change, and adaptation is a sign of resilience.
- **Learn from Challenges:** Embrace setbacks and challenges as learning opportunities. Use them to refine your approach and strengthen your commitment.

10. Patience and Persistence:

- **Stay Committed:** Holistic well-being is a lifelong journey. Stay committed to your goals even during periods of slow progress or setbacks.

- **Celebrate Perseverance:** Recognize the value of persistence and dedication in achieving lasting well-being.

By setting achievable goals and tracking your progress with intention and mindfulness, you empower yourself to make consistent, meaningful strides in your holistic well-being journey. Your goals serve as guiding stars on your path to greater resilience, inner peace, and holistic health.

Encouraging Holistic Practices in Daily Life

The true power of holistic stress management lies in its seamless integration into your daily routine. Here's how you can encourage and embrace holistic practices as a natural part of your daily life:

1. Morning Rituals:

- **Start Your Day Mindfully:** Begin your morning with a few moments of mindful breathing, meditation, or stretching. This sets a positive tone for the day ahead.
- **Healthy Breakfast:** Fuel your body with a balanced, nourishing breakfast that supports your energy levels and well-being.

2. Mindful Moments Throughout the Day:

- **Mini Breaks:** Take short breaks during your workday for deep breaths, brief stretches, or a moment of mindfulness. These micro-practices can refresh your mind.
- **Lunchtime Mindfulness:** Eat your lunch mindfully, savoring each bite. Avoid distractions like screens to focus on the nourishment.

3. Stress Reduction at Work:

- **Workspace Zen:** Create a workspace that promotes relaxation, with soothing colors, plants, or calming scents from essential oil diffusers.
- **Breath Breaks:** Whenever you feel stressed or overwhelmed, pause for a few rounds of deep, calming breaths to reset.

4. Mindful Movement and Exercise:

- **Daily Activity:** Integrate mindful movement into your daily routine. Whether it's a brief yoga session, a mindful walk, or Tai Chi, make it a habit.
- **Outdoor Connection:** Whenever possible, take your physical activities outdoors to connect with nature.

5. Holistic Nutrition:

- **Meal Planning:** Dedicate time for meal planning and preparation. Prioritize whole, unprocessed foods that nourish your body.
- **Mindful Eating:** Eat with awareness, savoring each bite. Avoid rushed or distracted meals.

6. Evening Tranquility:

- **Wind-Down Routine:** Establish an evening routine that promotes relaxation. This may include herbal tea, reading, or gentle stretches.
- **Digital Detox:** Limit screen time before bedtime to improve sleep quality.

7. Mindfulness Before Sleep:

- **Pre-Bed Meditation:** Incorporate a short meditation or gratitude practice before sleep to ease your mind.
- **Breathing Techniques:** Use calming breathwork techniques to prepare your body for restful sleep.

8. Weekly Reflection:

- **Weekly Check-Ins:** Dedicate time each week to reflect on your holistic practices, set new goals, and adjust your routine as needed.
- **Gratitude Journal:** Maintain a gratitude journal to cultivate a positive outlook on life.

9. Mindful Technology Use:

- **Screen Boundaries:** Set boundaries for technology use. Designate screen-free times and areas in your home.
- **Mindful Consumption:** Consume digital content mindfully, focusing on what truly enhances your well-being.

10. Community and Support:

- **Engage with Others:** Share your holistic journey with friends, family, or a like-minded community. This fosters a sense of connection and accountability.
- **Support System:** Lean on your support system during challenging times. They can provide encouragement and understanding.

11. Adapt and Embrace Change:

- **Flexibility:** Be flexible and open to adjusting your holistic practices as needed. Life is ever-changing, and adaptation is a sign of resilience.
- **Embrace Change:** View changes in your routine as opportunities for growth and exploration.

By weaving holistic practices seamlessly into your daily life, you transform them from occasional rituals into powerful tools for ongoing well-being. Remember that consistency is key, and over time, these practices will become second nature, contributing to your resilience, balance, and holistic health. Your daily life becomes a canvas for a vibrant and fulfilling journey towards well-being.

Inspiring Success Stories: Holistic Approaches to Stress Transformation

Real-life stories of individuals who have transformed their stress management with holistic approaches can serve as powerful inspiration on your own journey. Here are a few testimonials that highlight the impact of holistic practices:

1. Mary's Journey to Inner Peace

- *Mary* had struggled with chronic stress for years, leading to sleepless nights and overwhelming anxiety. She decided to explore holistic approaches and began a daily meditation practice. Over time, she noticed a profound shift in her well-being. Her anxiety reduced, and she experienced more restful sleep. Mary's journey inspired her to share mindfulness techniques with her family, creating a ripple effect of calm and positivity in her home.

2. John's Quest for Balance

- *John*, a busy professional, found himself constantly frazzled and disconnected from his well-being. He started practicing yoga and Tai Chi as a way to incorporate mindfulness into his life. Gradually, John felt a greater sense of balance and mental clarity. These practices not only helped him manage stress but also enhanced his focus and productivity at work. John's colleagues noticed the change and joined him in his mindful lunchtime stretches.

3. Emily's Aromatherapy Awakening

- *Emily* had always been intrigued by aromatherapy but had never explored it until she experienced a particularly stressful period in her life. She began using calming essential oils in her daily routine, from diffusing lavender at night to inhaling citrus scents during the day. Emily found that these scents not only reduced her stress but also uplifted her mood. She shared her newfound passion for aromatherapy with friends and even started crafting personalized blends for special occasions.

4. Mark's Herbal Healing

- *Mark* had been relying on prescription medication to manage his stress-related sleep issues for years. Concerned about the side effects, he consulted an herbalist who introduced him to adaptogenic herbs. With the guidance of the herbalist, Mark incorporated herbal teas and tinctures into his daily routine. Over time, he experienced more restful sleep without the need for medication. Mark's story encouraged his family members to explore herbal remedies for various health concerns.

5. Sarah's Nutritional Transformation

- *Sarah*, a mother of three, had a hectic lifestyle that often left her feeling drained and irritable. She decided to overhaul her family's diet, focusing on whole, nutritious foods. The impact was remarkable. Her family's energy levels increased, and they experienced fewer mood swings. Sarah's story of transformation inspired her friends to start meal planning and cooking together, strengthening their bond while prioritizing holistic nutrition.

These stories highlight the diverse ways in which holistic approaches can positively impact stress management and overall well-being. Each individual's journey is unique, but they all share a common theme: the power of holistic practices to bring balance, resilience, and inner peace. As you integrate holistic approaches into your life, remember that your own story of transformation is waiting to be written, filled with the potential for growth, healing, and holistic well-being.

A Plea for Reviews

Dear Readers and Friends,

I hope you've found "Holistic Approaches to Stress Management" to be a source of inspiration, guidance, and empowerment on your journey to a more balanced and stress-free life.

As an author, there's nothing more valuable than hearing from you, our cherished readers. Your feedback and reviews play a vital role in helping others discover the transformative power of holistic practices and well-being.

If this book has touched your life, provided you with practical tools, or resonated with your own experiences, please consider leaving a review. Your words can inspire others to embark on their own path to holistic well-being.

Your review doesn't need to be lengthy; even a few sentences sharing your thoughts, insights, or the impact the book has had on you can make a world of difference.

To post a review, simply visit the platform where you purchased the book and share your feedback.

Thank you for being a part of this journey toward greater resilience, vitality, and peace. Your reviews are not just words on a page; they are a way to pay it forward, helping others discover the path to holistic well-being.

With heartfelt gratitude,

Gabriella Goldberger

Don't miss out!

Visit the website below and you can sign up to receive emails whenever Gabriella Goldberger publishes a new book. There's no charge and no obligation.

https://books2read.com/r/B-A-CNJAB-WYVNC

BOOKS 2 READ

Connecting independent readers to independent writers.

www.ingramcontent.com/pod-product-compliance
Lightning Source LLC
Chambersburg PA
CBHW070839160726
48004CB00001B/433